Immunity in Viral and Rickettsial Diseases

ADVANCES IN EXPERIMENTAL MEDICINE AND BIOLOGY

Volume 1
THE RETICULOENDOTHELIAL SYSTEM AND ATHEROSCLEROSIS
Edited by N. R. Di Luzio and R. Paoletti • 1967

Volume 2
PHARMACOLOGY OF HORMONAL POLYPEPTIDES AND PROTEINS
Edited by N. Back, L. Martini, and R. Paoletti • 1968

Volume 3
GERM-FREE BIOLOGY: Experimental and Clinical Aspects
Edited by E. A. Mirand and N. Back • 1969

Volume 4
DRUGS AFFECTING LIPID METABOLISM
Edited by W. L. Holmes, L. A. Carlson, and R. Paoletti • 1969

Volume 5
LYMPHATIC TISSUE AND GERMINAL CENTERS IN IMMUNE RESPONSE
Edited by L. Fiore-Donati and M. G. Hanna, Jr. • 1969

Volume 6
RED CELL METABOLISM AND FUNCTION
Edited by George J. Brewer • 1970

Volume 7
SURFACE CHEMISTRY OF BIOLOGICAL SYSTEMS
Edited by Martin Blank • 1970

Volume 8
BRADYKININ AND RELATED KININS: Cardiovascular, Biochemical, and Neural Actions
Edited by F. Sicuteri, M. Rocha e Silva, and N. Back • 1970

Volume 9
SHOCK: Biochemical, Pharmacological, and Clinical Aspects
Edited by A. Bertelli and N. Back • 1970

Volume 10
THE HUMAN TESTIS
Edited by E. Rosemberg and C. A. Paulsen • 1970

Volume 11
MUSCLE METABOLISM DURING EXERCISE
Edited by B. Pernow and B. Saltin • 1971

Volume 12
MORPHOLOGICAL AND FUNCTIONAL ASPECTS OF IMMUNITY
Edited by K. Lindahl-Kiessling, G. Alm, and M. G. Hanna, Jr. • 1971

Volume 13
CHEMISTRY AND BRAIN DEVELOPMENT
Edited by R. Paoletti and A. N. Davison • 1971

Volume 14
MEMBRANE-BOUND ENZYMES
Edited by G. Porcellati and F. di Jeso • 1971

Volume 15
THE RETICULOENDOTHELIAL SYSTEM AND IMMUNE PHENOMENA
Edited by N. R. Di Luzio and K. Flemming • 1971

Volume 16A
THE ARTERY AND THE PROCESS OF ARTERIOSCLEROSIS: Pathogenesis
Edited by Stewart Wolf • 1971

Volume 16B
THE ARTERY AND THE PROCESS OF ARTERIOSCLEROSIS: Measurement and Modification
Edited by Stewart Wolf • 1972

Volume 17
CONTROL OF RENIN SECRETION
Edited by Tatiana A. Assaykeen • 1972

Volume 18
THE DYNAMICS OF MERISTEM CELL POPULATIONS
Edited by Morton W. Miller and Charles C. Kuehnert • 1972

Volume 19
SPHINGOLIPIDS, SPHINGOLIPIDOSES AND ALLIED DISORDERS
Edited by Bruno W. Volk and Stanley M. Aronson • 1972

Volume 20
DRUG ABUSE: Nonmedical Use of Dependence-Producing Drugs
Edited by Simon Btesh • 1972

Volume 21
VASOACTIVE POLYPEPTIDES
Edited by N. Back and F. Sicuteri • 1972

Volume 22
COMPARATIVE PATHOPHYSIOLOGY OF CIRCULATORY DISTURBANCES
Edited by Colin M. Bloor • 1972

Volume 23
THE FUNDAMENTAL MECHANISMS OF SHOCK
Edited by Lerner B. Hinshaw and Barbara G. Cox • 1972

Volume 24
THE VISUAL SYSTEM: Neurophysiology, Biophysics, and Their Clinical Applications
Edited by G. B. Arden • 1972

Volume 25
GLYCOLIPIDS, GLYCOPROTEINS, AND MUCOPOLYSACCHARIDES OF THE NERVOUS SYSTEM
Edited by Vittorio Zambotti, Guido Tettamanti, and Mariagrazia Arrigoni • 1972

Volume 26
PHARMACOLOGICAL CONTROL OF LIPID METABOLISM
Edited by William L. Holmes, Rodolfo Paoletti, and David Kritchevsky • 1972

Volume 27
DRUGS AND FETAL DEVELOPMENT
Edited by M. A. Klingberg, A. Abramovici, and J. Chemke • 1972

Volume 28
HEMOGLOBIN AND RED CELL STRUCTURE AND FUNCTION
Edited by George J. Brewer • 1972

Volume 29
MICROENVIRONMENTAL ASPECTS OF IMMUNITY
Edited by Branislav D. Janković and Katarina Isaković • 1972

Volume 30
HUMAN DEVELOPMENT AND THE THYROID GLAND: Relation to Endemic Cretinism
Edited by J. B. Stanbury and R. L. Kroc • 1972

Volume 31
IMMUNITY IN VIRAL AND RICKETTSIAL DISEASES
Edited by A. Kohn and M. A. Klingberg • 1972

Volume 32
FUNCTIONAL AND STRUCTURAL PROTEINS OF THE NERVOUS SYSTEM
Edited by A. N. Davison, P. Mandel, and I. G. Morgan • 1972

Immunity in Viral and Rickettsial Diseases

Proceedings of the Seventeenth Annual "OHOLO" Biological Conference on New Concepts in Immunity in Viral and Rickettsial Diseases Held March 13-16, 1972, at Zichron Yaakov, Israel

Edited by

Alexander Kohn

Director
Israel Institute for Biological Research, Ness-Ziona
Tel-Aviv University Medical School

and

Marcus A. Klingberg

Head
Department of Epidemiology
Israel Institute for Biological Research, Ness-Ziona
Tel-Aviv University Medical School

PLENUM PRESS • NEW YORK-LONDON • 1972

A Conference sponsored by the
ISRAEL INSTITUTE FOR BIOLOGICAL RESEARCH
Ness-Ziona, Israel

DOI 10.1007/978-1-4684-3225-1

MyCopy version of the original edition 1972

A Division of Plenum Publishing Corporation
227 West 17th Street, New York, N.Y. 10011

United Kingdom edition published by Plenum Press, London
A Division of Plenum Publishing Company
Davis House (4th Floor), 8 Scrubs Lane, Harlesden, London,
NW10 6SE, England

Organizing Committee:

PROF. ANDRE DE VRIES, Tel-Aviv University, Ramat-Aviv
PROF. NATAN GOLDBLUM, Hebrew University, Jerusalem
PROF. ROBERT GOLDWASSER, Israel Institute for Biological Research, Ness-Ziona
PROF. NATHAN GROSSOWICZ, Hebrew University, Jerusalem
MR. DAVID KATZ, Israel Institute for Biological Research, Ness-Ziona
PROF. ALEXANDER KEYNAN, Hebrew University, Jerusalem
PROF. ALEXANDER KOHN, Israel Institute for Biological Research, Ness-Ziona
PROF. MARCUS A. KLINGBERG, Israel Institute for Biological Research, Ness-Ziona

Secretary:
Mrs. Ilana Turner

PREFACE

The OHOLO conferences have been convened annually as from the spring of 1956; they have covered very wide areas from different and overlapping disciplines, as can be seen from the following list:

1956 Bacterial Genetics (not published)
1957 Tissue Cultures in Virological Research (not published)
1958 Inborn and Acquired Resistance to Infection in Animals (not published)
1959 Experimental Approach to Mental Diseases (not published)
1960 Cryptobiotic Stages in Biological Systems*
1961 Virus - Cell Relationships**
1962 Biological Synthesis and Function of Nucleic Acids**
1963 Cellular Control Mechanism of Macromolecular Synthesis**
1964 Molecular Aspects of Immunology**
1965 Cell Surfaces**
1966 Chemistry and Biology of Psychotropic Agents (not published)
1967 Structure and Mode of Action of Enzymes**
1968 Growth and Differentiation of Cells *in vitro***
1969 Behaviour of Animal Cells in Culture**
1970 Microbial Toxins**
1971 Interaction of Chemical Agents with Cholinergic Mechanisms**

The participants at these meetings from the different scientific institutions of Israel and from many countries, are engaged in fields of study which represent widely divergent approaches to biology. Thus, a characteristic feature of the OHOLO meetings has been their multi-disciplinary nature.

These small international conferences are distinguished by the relaxed atmosphere in which they are held, with ample time for informal as well as formal discussions.

*Published by Elsevier Publishing Co., Amsterdam (1960).
**Published by the Israel Institute for Biological Research, Ness-Ziona.

The present volume contains almost all the papers presented at the Seventeenth OHOLO Biological Conference, devoted to New Concepts in Immunity in Viral and Rickettsial Diseases, held at Zichron Yaakov, Israel, on March 13 - 16, 1972.

In order to obtain an overview of the broad spectrum of knowledge in this field and to review a considerable number of topics related to immunity in viral and rickettsial diseases, noted investigators have gathered together to analyze goals already achieved and speculate on the future potential for the prevention of viral and rickettsial diseases.

More than one hundred and sixty scientists (including twenty from overseas) participated in this meeting, and the eighteen papers presented summarized much data gathered in extensive laboratory, clinical and epidemiological studies.

For the success of our Symposium, we must thank the Chairman of the Sessions and the Moderator of the Round Table Discussion the participants who presented papers, and all those who joined in the discussions and so willingly cooperated in their contributing to this record of the Conference.

We believe that this Symposium provided an opportunity for the cross fertilization and stimulation of ideas between scientists in the various disciplines. The information gathered in this volume shows how much has already been done and what prospects lie ahead.

The meeting could not have been organized without the help of Mrs. Ilana Turner, Secretary of the Symposium, and Mr. Hanoch Yorav who helped with extracurricular tasks. Likewise, we are happy to thank the secretaries, Mmes. Rachel Straks, Janina Gittelman and Nita Ben-David for their tireless efforts on our behalf.

The Editors gladly take this opportunity to express their thanks to the Organizing Committee for their efforts and dedication in preparing the meeting, and gratefully acknowledge the efficient assistance of Mrs. Myra Kaye in editing and Mrs. LaVerne Binstock in the technical preparation of the manuscript for publication.

Alexander Kohn

Marcus A. Klingberg

CONTENTS

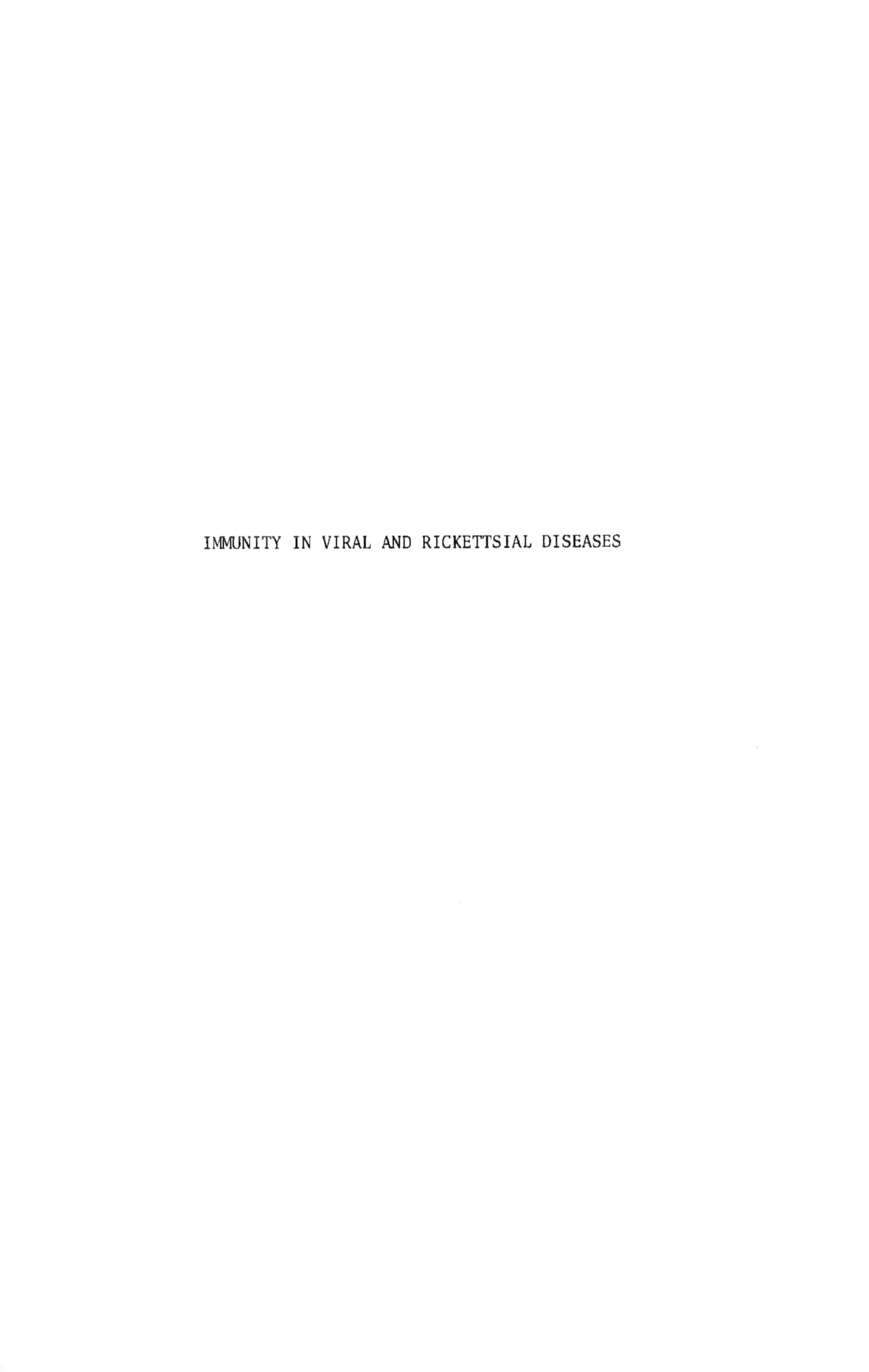

IMMUNITY IN VIRAL AND RICKETTSIAL DISEASES

WELCOMING ADDRESS

Alexander Kohn

Israel Institute for Biological Research

Ness-Ziona, Israel

I have pleasure in opening this 17th "OHOLO" conference on "New Concepts in Immunology of Viral and Rickettsial Diseases". We are very flattered that some of our distinguished colleagues found the time and means to come here from all parts of the globe in order to share with us their experience and knowledge. On behalf of myself and the Israel Institute for Biological Research, which organized this meeting, I extend our heartiest welcome to you all.

There is a certain incongruity between the name of the conference - the "OHOLO CONFERENCE" - and the fact that it takes place in Zikhron Yaakov. During the past 16 years, the OHOLO meetings were indeed held at Oholo, on the shores of the Lake of Galilee, 14 times. For reasons beyond our control, this year we have had to alter our venue and hold the conference here.

It is proper, however, to devote a few words to the concept of the OHOLO conferences and to OHOLO itself:

OHOLO is an educational institution, operated by an autonomous unit of the Cultural Center of the Histadrut (General Federation of Labour). It was established by Ben-Zion Israeli, a member of the Kibbutz Kinereth, in memory of Berl Katzenelson, founder and editor of the Histadrut's daily newspaper DAVAR, and one of the leaders of the Zionist socialist movement. The word OHOLO means "his tent", based on the expression "Ohel Tora" - the place where the Tora (Bible) is taught.

The OHOLO conferences were originated by Prof. A. Keynan, the late Prof. S. Hestrin and Prof. N. Grossowicz of the Hebrew University, Jerusalem. They are organized by the Israel Institute for Biological Research at Ness-Ziona, an institute under the aegis of the Prime Minister's Office,which is engaged in basic and applied research in the clinical and experimental epidemiology of bacterial, viral and fungal disease; and in the fields of entomology and insecticides and of pharmacological chemistry.

The purpose of the OHOLO meetings is to foster interdisciplinary communication in biology between Israeli scientists and their colleagues abroad. The topics discussed at these conferences have included, among others, genetics, virology, immunology, cell biology, embryology, psychotropic agents, mental diseases and microbial toxins.

Immunology as well as virology are rapidly advancing fields in the biological sciences. Immunization is still the only generally effective means of preventing viral infection in animals. And the beginnings of both virology and immunology are interlinked in the investigations of Jenner. It is interesting to note that Jenner, despite his erroneous concepts concerning the etiology of smallpox and cowpox (he actually believed cowpox was a horse disease due to grease affecting the heels) was, at a time when nobody knew anything about bacteria and viruses, so successful in initiating a vaccination procedure against smallpox which holds good to this very day. Jenner's vaccination procedure contributed to the virtual disappearance of classical smallpox from Europe during the 19th century, and today there remain only eight countries in the whole world where smallpox still occurs.

Since I am interested in the epidemic spread of obscurantism in science, I should like to use this opportunity to quote from Jenner's treatise "An Inquiry into the Causes and Effects of the Variolae Vaccinae, etc.":

> "Thus far have I proceeded in an enquiry founded, as it must appear, on the basis of experiment; in which, however, conjecture has been occasionally admitted in order to present to persons well situated for such discussions objects for more minute investigations."

Now, in contrast to the times of Jenner, in this second half of the 20th century, when our knowledge of virology has mushroomed to the extent that there is already a whole 800 page book just on lambda phage, we are still quite far from a successful and foolproof control of viral diseases. In the field with which we are concerned at this conference, the immunology of viral and rickettsial diseases, there are still many problems unsolved. Just to name some - the difficulty of cultivating certain viruses in sufficient quantity; how to deal with viruses possessing many antigenically different strains; uncertainties as to duration of immunity; criteria for comparative efficacy of vaccine purification and fractionation with retention of immunogenicity; live versus killed vaccines; the relative importance of interferon and delayed hypersensitivity; and there are many others. In this short meeting we are going to be able to discuss only some of these problems.

I should like to end by quoting from Paul Ehrlich, whose remarks in his Berben Lecture in London in 1908 are still relevant for us today:

> "It is our task to advance by a more accurate and more extensive study of all the haptines and their actions, and in the first place we must gain a knowledge of the influence exerted upon the causes of infection by the distribution and action of dissolved substances whose action is cytotropic, so that we may obtain a nearer insight into the manifold secondary phenomena which arise from them."

I end with the hope that the flames of our discussions will produce more light than smoke and that everyone will thoroughly enjoy his stay here.

VIRUSES AND THE IMMUNE RESPONSE

Frank Fenner

John Curtin School of Medical Research
Australian National University
Canberra, Australia

HISTORICAL ASPECTS

There have been close links between the development of virology and that of immunology for a very long time. One could say that they were born together in 1798, when Edward Jenner introduced vaccination with cowpox to protect against the smallpox. Contained within this discovery were the recognition of a contagious viral disease, an appreciation of cross-reactivity between related viruses and the notions of active immunization and delayed hypersensitivity. Almost a century later, Louis Pasteur deliberately attenuated virulent rabies virus by serial passage in a novel host, the rabbit, thus introducing a method of preparing live virus vaccines that persists to the present day. More recently, it was primarily the consideration of Traub's experiments with congenital lymphocytic choriomeningitis of mice that led in 1949 to Burnet's concept of immunological tolerance; and it was Burnet's experience as a microbiologist, thinking of the genetics of viruses and bacteria as exercises in population genetics, that led him to a similar consideration of lymphoid cell populations and the enunciation of the clonal selection theory of antibody production in 1959.

We get a good idea of the state of virology and immunology in 1959 by consulting two books published about that time; the second edition of Burnet's "Principles of Animal Virology" (1960), and the third edition of Rivers and Horsfall "The Viral and Rickettsial Infections of Man." We find immunology at that time largely dominated by the consideration of serum antibodies, primarily antibodies to soluble proteins, with a few "non-conformists" battling with the significance of delayed hypersensitivity, as exemplified by the tuberculin response; and fewer still, primarily Medawar and his colleagues, experimenting with the immunology of graft rejection. At the level of the organism, virology was concerned almost entirely with acute infections, although the introduction of tissue culture for diagnostic virology a decade earlier had uncovered a host of "viruses in search of disease" -- the orphan viruses -- and was beginning to force home the fact that all animals and most cultured cells harbored latent viruses. Chemical virology, with viruses other than tobacco mosaic virus, was still at the developmental state, struggling with techniques for purification, separation and characterization of viruses and their components. Since negative staining for electron microscopy of viruses was not introduced until 1959 we were then restricted in our concepts of viral structure to the crude pictures obtained with a few viruses using shadowed preparations and thin sections.

My next dateline for assessing the progress of virology and immunology is 1967, when I completed writing a successor to Burnet's "Principles of Animal Virology," called "The Biology of Animal Viruses." By then there had been a very substantial change in the outlook and the content of virology and immunology. The tissue culture revolution was complete and experiments in cultured cells dominated the virologic scene -- as they have ever since. In immunology, cellular and transplantation immunology shared honors with detailed chemical analysis of the structure of immunoglobulins as the main growing edges; and in virology study of the tumor viruses had become a lusty youngster, making up in its speed of growth for a prolonged gestation, for it had been conceived by Rous in 1911. The principle fruits of the negative staining method had been reaped, and our mental pictures of viruses were changed for all time by its revelations. The difficulties of synchronized infection of cultured cells had largely been overcome and biochemical virology was beginning to reap a rich harvest -- the virions of a few viruses, like the adenoviruses for example, were being dissected into their constituent polypeptide and nucleic acid molecules and viral antigens were being conceived in molecular terms rather than as titers in serological tests. At the levels of cell and organism,fluorescent antibody staining had provided a powerful way of localizing viral multiplication in the cell and in the animal body. An increasing number of virologists were turning their attention to persistent viruses and latent infections. Kuru had just been transmitted to chimpanzees, and hypotheses about the viral etiology of chronic degenerative diseases of the central nervous system in man received their first experimental support.

Looking at the areas of contact of virology and immunology in 1967, as I then saw the field, the concept of local immunity and secretory immunoglobulins found a place, as did the notion that immune responses were sometimes responsible for the pathological results associated with viral infection. Cellular immune responses were considered primarily in relation to tumor rejection, and it was still orthodox in 1967 to look on lymphocytic choriomeningitis of mice as a completely tolerated infection.

Since then the information explosion has continued at an accelerated pace. It is said that the volume of scientific literature doubles every 15 years. Both virology and immunology are growing much more rapidly than this. As an illustration I present some figures taken from a selection of English language journals specifically in those fields, for the three years that I mentioned previously - 1960, 1967 and 1971. For immunology, the annual page numbers went from 1,700 to 6,700 to 12,300 pages; for virology, from 2,500 to 5,000 to 8,000 pages.

THE OHOLO CONFERENCE

So much for the past. I have given you a greatly compressed outline of the movements that led up to our present Oholo Conference, "New Concepts of Immunity in Viral and Rickettsial Disease." Very briefly, and without anticipating their content, I shall sketch the scope of the Conference and the nature of the papers that we shall hear. I shall then conclude by looking in somewhat greater depth at some aspects of the immunology of viral infections not covered by the symposium.

The Definition of Viral Antigens

As far as immunization is concerned, it is clearly useful to define just what viral antigens are important for protection. Advances in biochemical techniques of separation and purification of macromolecules are now making it possible to describe the polypeptides of virus particles quite precisely, although this work is limited by the difficulties of scale that virologists are familiar with, but some of our biochemical colleagues don't understand. And perhaps virologists also do not think on a large enough scale. I was struck the other day, in conversation with a very astute biochemist, with the importance of scaling up operations if one is to do meaningful biochemistry. He told me how his attitude to these matters had been affected by the opening sentences of papers by those great German biochemists, Warburg and Butenandt, who used as starting material for the isolation of rare substances "the blood of 5000 horses," for pyridine nucleotide; "half ton of yeast" for lumiflavin, and tank-car quantities of human male urine for androsterone.

The four papers set for tomorrow morning are devoted to specific aspects of this problem -- i.e., viral antigens -- and on Wednesday Drs. Pereira and Arnon will address themselves to the questions that will arise if and when virologists do completely define which viral antigens are important for protection; "Are vaccines of purified proteins practicable (from the point of view of production), and will they work?" and "Can we look beyond the isolation of viral antigens to the deliberate synthesis of the relevant antigenic determinants?"

The Host Response in Vaccination

Clearly, effective immunization depends on achieving an appropriate immune-response -- appropriate in terms of the potency and amount of antibody, the time course of its production, the potential for recall, and the location of antibody in relation to its capacity to influence key points in the pathogenesis of viral infection. Here the most important lessons of the last few years relate to that aspect of protection that Dr. Sabin emphasized so vigorously fifteen years ago, when he talked of 'gut immunity' in poliomyelitis, namely the production of secretory immunoglobulins on the great mucous surfaces through which so many viruses gain entry to the body, or cause disease by multiplying locally. The Conference is fortunate in having Dr. Waldman to address us on this important topic. My own technical paper will be concerned with virological aspects of the same problem, since much of the pressure to develop new viral vaccines derives from the need to control respiratory infections, and the respiratory tract provides a temperature gradient that can be exploited with temperature-sensitive mutants. Then, since antibody production is under genetic control, we must look at the possibility that some "antigens" may not function in particular animals for genetical reasons. This is an area in which Dr. Sela's group at Rehovoth has been a pioneer.

The Production of Viral Vaccines

Given that we understand what is needed, virologically, and know how to introduce it so as to produce the desired immune response, we come to the problem of producing the vaccine. With viruses and rickettsiae, vaccine production presents problems not faced by those concerned with bacterial vaccines -- not only the problem of scaling up that I mentioned earlier but the fact that one must use a cell substrate; and there are many who now believe that no cell exists that does not carry at least one latent and potentially harmful virus. Most of Wednesday morning will be devoted to various aspects of this problem.

Immunity in the Individual and the Population

Finally, the Conference will consider the goal, or goals, of immunization. On the one hand the physician who treats individual patients is rightly concerned with what he should do to protect each individual. If every individual were adequately protected then the population as a whole would be protected, but in the real world, especially the larger and less affluent part of it, we can be sure that every individual will not be protected by the efforts of individual physicians. Our studies of the epidemiology of infectious diseases show that this is not necessary. The survival of viruses in nature depends on a variety of factors that includes as an important component, very different with different viruses, the size and turnover rate of the susceptible host population. If there is one regret that I have in surveying the excellent program prepared for us, it is that we shall not hear about the problems associated with the attempts to eradicate measles from the United States of America by vaccination, for measles provides better data than any other human disease on the population factors involved in the survival of the virus.

Rickettsial Infections

If in my preview of the topics to be covered in the Conference I have failed to mention rickettsial diseases, it is not because of a lack of interest in them, for the first paper I ever wrote in experimental biology related to North Queensland tick typhus. Rickettsial diseases do not now present the public health problems that they did in the past, though Dr. Wisseman will remind us that they have by no means disappeared. Even that symbol of misery and poverty, louse-borne typhus, could undergo a resurgence if social conditions worsen, as they have in the last few years in Biafra and Bangla Desh, for example. We shall hear from Dr. Wisseman about the prospects for using a live attenuated vaccine for the control of louse-borne typhus.

So much, then, for a glance at the historical development of virology and immunology and at the subjects for discussion over the next few days. Now I shall turn briefly to two other aspects of viral immunology, viz., the role of cell-mediated immunity in recovery from viral infections; and antibodies and complement in infections with persistent or recurrent viremia.

Cell-Mediated Immunity in Viral Infections

Protection against infection afforded by vaccination operates primarily through the humoral arm of the immune response. Less attention has been paid to the role of the immune response in recovery from primary viral infections, in the inhibition of viral growth and in sterilization of infectious foci, partly because antibody seemed so often to be an obvious mechanism. However, although antibody has a dramatic effect when injected during the incubation period of measles, for instance, this cannot be accepted as evidence that antibody always plays an important part during the natural recovery process. The role of cell-mediated immunity has not been studied in the past because of technical difficulties in measuring the cell-mediated immune response, and distinguishing it from antibodies. The discovery of interferon as an important antiviral factor made the problem even more difficult because a distinction now needs to be made between antibody, cell-mediated immunity and interferon.

Some evidence about the roles of antibody and cell-mediated immunity in recovery from viral infections is provided by certain "experiments of nature" in the form of patients in whom either the antibody or the cell-mediated immune response is deficient. Patients with agammaglobulinaemia fail to produce immunoglobulins but their cell-mediated immune response is usually not disturbed. The response to smallpox vaccination and to most viral infections is normal. Patients with thymic aplasia, in contrast, generally show normal antibody responses but fail to develop cell-mediated immunity, and in children suffering from this deficiency smallpox vaccination results in a progressive enlargement of the primary skin lesion that is unaffected by the administration of immune γ globulin. The defective cellular immune response in these patients is reflected in their inability to control certain fungal infections, and even administration of BCG vaccine has led to fatal systemic tuberculosis.

Experiments by Allison with fibroma virus in rabbits provide evidence of the separate roles of humoral antibodies and cell-mediated immunity in the pathogenesis of this viral infection. Treatment of adult rabbits with methotrexate suppressed both the humoral and the cell-mediated immune response, and the reaction of the rabbits to fibroma virus was then modified in two ways: generalized fibromatosis developed and the regression of individual tumors was greatly delayed. Large doses of immune serum prevented generalization by suppressing viremia, but had no effect on the rate of regression. Cortisone treatment impaired the development of cell-mediated immunity more than it affected the production of antibodies; cortisone-treated rabbits did not get generalized fibromatosis but regression of the tumors that developed at the inoculation site was greatly delayed. These observations, and the regular occurrence of large numbers of mononuclear cells in normal regressing fibromas coupled with their absence from the persistent fibromas of immunosuppressant-treated rabbits, suggest strongly that regression of these virus-induced tumors is due to a cell-mediated immune response.

Recently Blanden, working in Canberra, has provided more conclusive evidence for the role of cell-mediated immunity in recovery from certain viral infections. First, he showed that mice infected with sublethal doses of ectromelia virus died if they were treated with antilymphocytic serum, apparently as a result of the uncontrolled growth of virus in the liver. The antilymphocytic serum suppressed the cell-mediated immune response, but not the antibody or interferon responses. He then transferred splenic lymphocytes to mice infected one day earlier with ectromelia virus, and found that immune but not normal lymphocytes caused a striking inhibition of viral growth and a fall in viral titer in target organs. This effect was demonstrable within 24 hours of cell transfer, and was greatly reduced if the transfused cells were treated with anti-lumphocytic serum, anti-θ (thymus-derived cell antigen) serum, or anti-light chain serum. In these experiments the recipients of the immune cells did not develop detectable antibody, although when hyperimmune mouse serum was transfused, high titer antibody was found in the recipients, inhibition of further viral growth, but no fall in viral titer. Passively transferred interferon had no effect on viral titers. Thus thymus-derived lymphocytes are probably the primary agents of the antiviral effect, which was accompanied by an infiltration of lymphocytes and monocytes into liver lesions. There appeared to be a requirement for a radiation-sensitive host component, probably a bone-marrow derived macrophage, for the full expression of the antiviral effect.

Sensitized lymphocytes exert their antiviral effects in several ways. First, by liberating lymphokines on exposure to antigens in tissues, they induce the migration and activation of macrophages. These macrophages, perhaps with the help of small amounts of antibody or locally produced interferon, phagocytose and digest infected material. Second, sensitized lymphocytes encountering intact infected cells that bear viral antigens on their surface, can kill such cells before virus is liberated; an obvious mechanism for inhibiting budding viruses, but probably important in many other situations, including the case of ectromelia referred to above. Third, sensitized lymphocytes may liberate interferon on exposure to antigen, and this could have a significant antiviral effect in tissues.

Thus, cell-mediated immunity plays a central role in recovery from at least some viral infections. The evidence, however, relates to certain systemic infections, primarily those with cell-associated rather than a plasma-associated viremia. Other recovery mechanisms are probably more important in viral infections of epithelial surfaces. For instance, antilymphocytic serum, which depresses cell-mediated immunity, has no detectable effect on the pathogenicity for mice of intranasally infused influenza virus, or Sendai virus, suggesting that antibodies or interferon are more important in these cases. Further, agammaglobulinaemic children, with normal cell-mediated immunity, showed increased susceptibility to oral infection with poliovirus. It is not only neutralizing antibodies that may be important in host resistance. Antibody directed against any viral antigen present in infected tissues could, by forming immune complexes, induce the inflammatory infiltrates that lead to an antiviral effect. Probably antibody, cell-mediated immunity and interferon each play a part in recovery from all viral infections, although in different situations one of these factors may be much more important than the others.

PERSISTENT VIRAL INFECTIONS

We now know of a great variety of situations in which viral infection persists long after the initial attack, either latent, or with continued viral expression.

Subacute Spongiform Encephalopathies

The subacute spongiform viral encephalopathies comprise scrapie, mink encephalopathy, kuru and Creutzfeld-Jacob disease, in all of which the incubation period lasts for years, and disease, once evident, progresses slowly and inevitably to death. These diseases are unique immunologically in that at no time in their prolonged course is there the slightest indication of an immune response, humoral or cellular. The difficulty in studying these diseases illustrates just how much the investigator depends upon and uses the immune response for the analysis of viruses and viral infections. It also emphasizes the curious nature of the scrapie agent -- a replicating fragment of genetic information that is filterable but is very resistant to heat, formalin and radiation; and is non-antigenic. Perhaps the best guess as to its nature is that the "virus" is a small piece of nucleic acid, perhaps no heavier than 100,000 daltons, that is protected from nucleases and inactivation by physical agents by a close association with membranes. There is a precedent for this in the plant virus, the potato spindle tuber virus, that has been studied by Dr. Diener.

Herpesvirus Infections

In these classic latent infections, herpes simplex and varicella-zoster, there is now good experimental evidence to suggest that latency is due to persistence of the virus in an occult form in the neuronal cells of the spinal ganglion. It is unlikely to be an integrated genome because these cells do not multiply; perhaps it persists as a repressed episome. When multiplication is triggered the virus moves by multiplication and infection down the Schwann cells of the sensory nerve trunks to the appropriate area of skin. There is some evidence, but not conclusive, that recurrence may be related to a falling antibody level. If so the mechanism is puzzling, because of the protected intracellular site of the virus both in the ganglion and during its passage down the nerve trunk.

Circulating Virus-Antibody Complexes

Finally, there are several diseases of mice in which viremia seems to persist for the normal or perhaps a somewhat shorter lifespan span of the mouse. I refer to murine leukemia, lactic dehydrogenase virus infection and lymphocytic choriomeningitis of mice. Here we find that the infection is often congenital, but in contrast to our earlier belief, immunological tolerance is at best partial. True, free circulating antibody is difficult to demonstrate, but the viremia consists of circulatory virus-antibody complexes, many of which are infectious. To varying extents in the different diseases these complexes have complement associated with them, and are deposited in the tissues to cause glomerulonephritis and vasculitis, which may be the principal causes of disease and death.

DENGUE SHOCK SYNDROME

I will turn from these persistent infections to a very interesting example of recurrent infection that has produced a "new" disease and that has important implications in relation to future vaccination programs. This is the disease called "dengue shock syndrome" or "dengue hemorrhagic fever." Hemorrhagic skin lesions were recognized as a very rare complication of the epidemics of dengue that recurrently swept this part of the world, Australia and southeast Asia. But in 1954 hemorrhagic fever appeared to be much more common than ever before in outbreaks of dengue in the Phillipines, and subsequently it has become common in Thailand, India and elsewhere. At first there appeared to be an ethnic component -- Chinese and Caucasians were thought not to get the disease. Now we know that dengue hemorrhagic fever is an immunological disease. There are four serotypes of dengue virus that cross-react by complement fixation but do not confer a high lever of cross-protection. There is nevertheless a rapid serological response when an individual who has recovered from an attack of dengue due to one serotype is infected with another. The secondary antibody response coincides with viremia due to the super-infecting dengue virus and in a proportion of individuals circulatory immune complexes are formed and complement depletion occurs. The immune complexes deposit in vessel walls and hemorrhagic fever and shock result. The apparent "ethnic component" reflected the higher incidence of second attacks of dengue, with different serotypes, in Thais rather than Caucasians or Chinese.

Why has dengue hemorrhagic fever now appeared as a 'new disease' in so many countries in south and southeast Asia? It appears to be due to the particular and novel social conditions that are developing. *Aedes aegypti*, the major vector of dengue, is enzootic throughout the area. In the past, when most people remained for most of the time in their own villages, there was endemic dengue and an occasional epidemic when a new serotype was introduced. Now, with the great social mobility that is characteristic of these parts of the world since World War II, infection with several serotypes of dengue virus is constantly and almost universally endemic, so that there are many second infections with different serotypes. In a proportion of these, the antibody response is such that circulating virus-antibody-complement complexes are formed, and the dengue shock syndrome results. It is important for public health officials to recognize that in populations like this, vaccination against dengue might well set the stage for more cases of this severe complication, a result that would hardly compensate for lowering the incidence of mild dengue.

UNRESOLVED PROBLEMS

Finally, let me list some unsolved problems that those concerned with vaccines will have to give thought to in the future. Firstly, where do we stop? Hundreds of different viruses cause human disease of greater or lesser severity. We have now got effective vaccines against many of the serious generalized infections -- how far can we expect to go in providing vaccines against the host of respiratory infections that characterize modern urban life? Secondly, there is the practical problem of keeping up vaccination when diseases all but disappear. With smallpox, where vaccination itself carries a small but real risk, many countries have now decided to stop vaccinating their citizens, and demanding vaccination certificates from visitors to their countries. A more difficult situation is that found in poliomyelitis and perhaps may soon be found in measles, where people have stopped bringing their children in for vaccination, because the diseases seem to have disappeared. It may be that vaccination certificates against poliovirus and measles rather than against smallpox should be demanded of incoming travellers, in an attempt to minimize the importation of virulent strains of these viruses. Thirdly, how does our new knowledge of oncogenic viruses and chronic viral diseases like subacute sclerosing panencephalitis affect our attitude to vaccination, particularly if we introduce viral nucleic acids by the parenteral route? And finally, what about vaccines against cancer, if a "causative agent" turns out to be a virus that is carried in the genome of all individuals of the species involved?

Quite apart from the problems that we shall be discussing in the Conference over the next few days, this brief group of unanswered questions shows that there are several major challenges ahead for those who work on viral vaccines, which means that it will remain a scientifically interesting field as well as one of great practical importance for many years to come.

ACKNOWLEDGEMENT

This paper was prepared while the author was a Fogarty Scholar-in-Residence, Fogarty International Center, N.I.H.

STRUCTURE-FUNCTION RELATIONSHIPS IN FOOT-AND-MOUTH DISEASE VIRUS

F. Brown

Animal Virus Research Institute

Pirbright, Surrey, England

Foot-and-mouth disease is undoubtedly the most troublesome virus disease of farm livestock. Cattle, pigs, sheep and goats are all susceptible and the economic importance of these animals makes foot-and-mouth disease a problem which is considerable and of world-wide concern. At present the disease is combatted mainly by vaccination and some idea of the problem may be obtained from the knowledge that more than 1,000 million doses of vaccine are administered each year.

Foot-and-mouth disease virus occurs as seven distinct immunological types: O, A, C, SAT 1, SAT 2, SAT 3 and Asia 1. The degree of difference between these types is such that an animal which has recovered from infection with one type is still fully susceptible to the others, although it is immune to re-infection with virus of the same type. Besides the seven major types, however, sub-types exist within each type. These were originally defined as sub-types because, although belonging to the same general immunological group, they did not confer solid immunity in cross-immunity tests, i.e., a proportion of the animals were not immune to challenge with another sub-type within the type.

The multiplicity of virus types and sub-types means that the individual viruses have differences which must be reflected in their structure. They also differ in other respects as a consequence of their different structures. To cite one example, it is well established that inactivated vaccines prepared from some viruses have disturbingly low potency. It was not known until recently whether this was due to the lack of antigenic mass in the vaccines or to some qualitative difference in the structure of the poor vaccine strains. We now know that the difference between a good vaccine and a poor vaccine depends in large part on the stability of the immunizing antigen during inactivation and within the inoculated animals (1). The structural features underlying the difference in stability of good and poor vaccines are not known with certainty but it seems reasonable to expect that a study of the structure of the immunizing antigen will eventually reveal the reasons for this difference. During the last few years, we have been engaged on a study of the structure of foot-and-mouth disease virus with the aim of correlating the structural features of the virus with its biological properties, particularly with regard to the production of neutralizing antibody. Some of the results of this study are presented below.

Foot-and-mouth disease virus is a member of the picornavirus group. Apart from vesicular exanthema virus and the feline picornaviruses, this group has a rather uninteresting morphology (Fig. 1). All the viruses are roughly spherical but foot-and-mouth disease virus, with a diameter of 24 nm., is rather smaller than the other members of the group. The virus sediments at 140S, compared with 160S for poliovirus. Foot-and-mouth disease virus has a greater density in caesium chloride than most of the other members of the group. The buoyant density of 1.43 g/ml compares with a value of 1.34 g/ml for poliovirus and 1.40 g/ml for the rhinoviruses. There appears to be some relationship between the stability of the virus particles at pH's below 7 and their density in caesium chloride. Thus, poliovirus is stable at pH 3, whereas foot-and-mouth disease virus is unstable at pH values as high as 6.5.

From the small number of analyses which have been made, it appears that, in accordance with the other picornaviruses, foot-and-mouth disease virus contains 30 percent RNA and 70 percent protein. The RNA is present as one single strand of molecular weight 2.6×10^6, whereas the protein is made up of at least four polypeptides with molecular weights ranging from 34×10^3 to 13.5×10^3. The molecular weight of the RNA has been estimated from sedimentation data and by polyacrylamide gel electrophoresis. The well known hazards which are present in estimating the molecular weight of RNA from sedimentation data invite caution in stating an exact value for the molecular weight of the virus RNA. However, by using the method of Fenwick (2) in which the RNA is treated with formaldehyde to minimize configurational restraints before centrifuging in sucrose gradients, Newman (3) has found that the sedimentation coefficient of foot-and-mouth disease virus RNA is the same as that of encephalomyocarditis virus RNA, for which values of 2.4 to 2.7×10^6 have been obtained by physical and chemical methods. Since the RNA comprises 31 percent of the virus particle (4), the molecular weight of the virus is

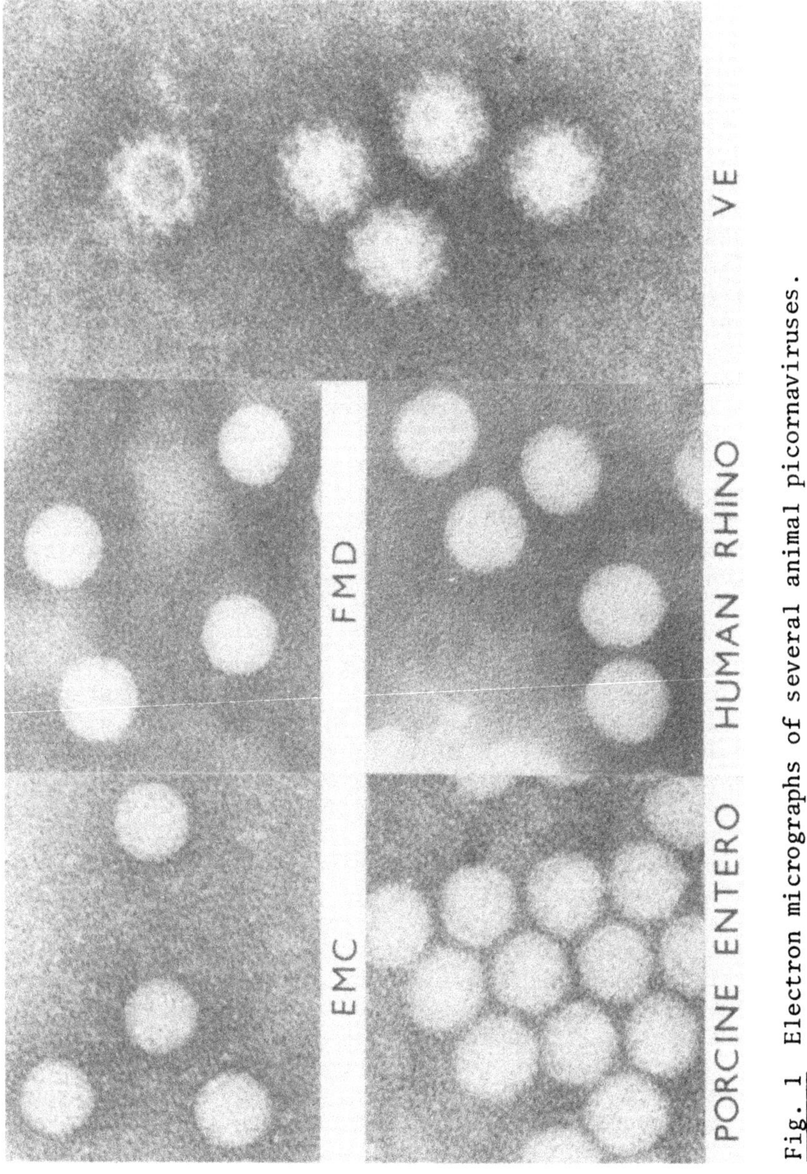

Fig. 1 Electron micrographs of several animal picornaviruses.

$2.6 \times 10^6 \times \frac{100}{31} = 8.4 \times 10^6$, of which the protein contributes 5.8×10^6.

Polyacrylamide gel electrophoresis of the viral polypeptides in the presence of sodium dodecyl sulphate shows the presence of four polypeptides with molecular weights of $10^3 \times 34$ (VP_1), 30 (VP_2), 26 (VP_3) and 13.5 (VP_4) (5). These polypeptides are present in the ratio 1 : 1 : 1 : 0.5, which is similar to the proportions found for several of the picornaviruses. As mentioned above, foot-and-mouth disease virus is unstable below pH 7, being dissociated into the virus RNA, a protein sub-unit consisting of the three larger polypeptides (VP_1, VP_2, VP_3) and an insoluble aggregate containing the smallest polypeptide, VP_4 (6). Strohmaier (7) and Liebermann and Schulze (8) estimated the molecular weight of the 12S sub-unit to be 289×10^3 and 282×10^3, respectively from its sedimentation coefficient and diffusion constant and we have obtained a value of 265×10^3 by electrophoresis in polyacrylamide gels (5). The molecular weights of the three polypeptides comprising the 12S sub-unit are 34, 30 and 26×10^3 and, as they are present in equimolar proportions, the monomeric unit will have a molecular weight of 90×10^3. This is compatible with the 12S sub-unit being a trimer with a molecular weight of 270×10^3.

A molecular weight of 5.8×10^6 for the protein of the virus would be in accordance with the presence of twenty 12S sub-units (total molecular weight 5.4×10^6) and thirty molecules of VP_4 (total molecular weight 0.41×10^6). The twenty 12S sub-units probably represent the triangular faces of the virus particle but the role of VP_4 is not known with any certainty.

Only the 140S particle possesses significant immunizing activity. The natural 12S particle, which is present in unfractionated virus harvests, and the artificial 12S particle obtained by mild acid disruption of the 140S particle produce less than one percent of the neutralizing antibody obtained by inoculation of an equal weight of 140S particles. The so-called empty 75S particles (9) produce as much neutralizing antibody as the full 140S particles, provided they are fixed with formaldehyde before inoculation (10). The immunizing activity of the 140S particles is closely associated with VP_1, since incubation with trypsin considerably reduces their immunizing activity. The polypeptide VP_1 is cleaved, leaving a smaller unit of molecular weight 19×10^3 (6), whereas the other polypeptides are apparently unaffected.

Electron microscopy of virus antibody complexes indicates that the trypsin-sensitive polypeptide is at the vertices of the particle (11), whereas IgG reacts with the entire surface of the virus particle, producing complexes in which the outline of the virus particles is obscure. IgM, or IgG which has been absorbed with 12S sub-units or trypsin-treated virus, forms complexes in which attachment is at regularly spaced sites on the virus surface (Figs. 2-4). Trypsin-treated virus also forms complexes of this type with IgG absorbed with 12S sub-units (Fig. 5). The virus thus appears to possess at least three types of combining sites, one on the faces of the particle and the others at regularly spaced intervals, probably at the vertices. IgM does not react with trypsin-treated virus particles in immunodiffusion or neutralization tests, indicating a higher degree of specificity for this class of antibody.

We have found recently that, in addition to the immunogenic site which is removed by trypsin, the virus particles contain a second site which can stimulate the production of neutralizing antibody. This was shown by the observation that trypsin-treated particles, although less potent than the intact particles, nevertheless produced significant amounts of neutralizing antibody. This antibody could be absorbed with trypsin-treated particles, whereas the virus-neutralizing activity of antiserum produced by inoculation of intact particles was unaffected by absorption with trypsin-treated particles. However, the activity of virus antiserum in neutralizing trypsin-treated particles was removed by absorption with trypsin-treated particles, showing that both antibodies are present in virus antisera.

The virus-neutralizing antibody appears to be concerned with preventing attachment of the virus to susceptible cells. However, the antibody produced by inoculating trypsin-treated particles does not prevent attachment. It is tempting to speculate that the role of this antibody is concerned with the uncoating process but we have no evidence at present to support such a view.

Despite the better understanding of the biological activities of the virus which has accrued from a detailed study of its structure, many problems remain unsolved. While we now know that VP_1 has an important role in producing immunity and that it is located at the vertices of the particle, our knowledge of the role of the other polypeptides is negligible. From the practical viewpoint of vaccination, retention of the integrity of the 140S particle is essential. Nevertheless, the factors determining the stability of the particle are unknown. It presumably depends on the interrelationship between the RNA and the polypeptides and on the stability of the bonds between the individual polypeptides themselves. These problems are almost completely unexplored. Investigation of these areas will provide valuable and worthwhile information on the structure of the virus and would also have considerable practical application in vaccine production.

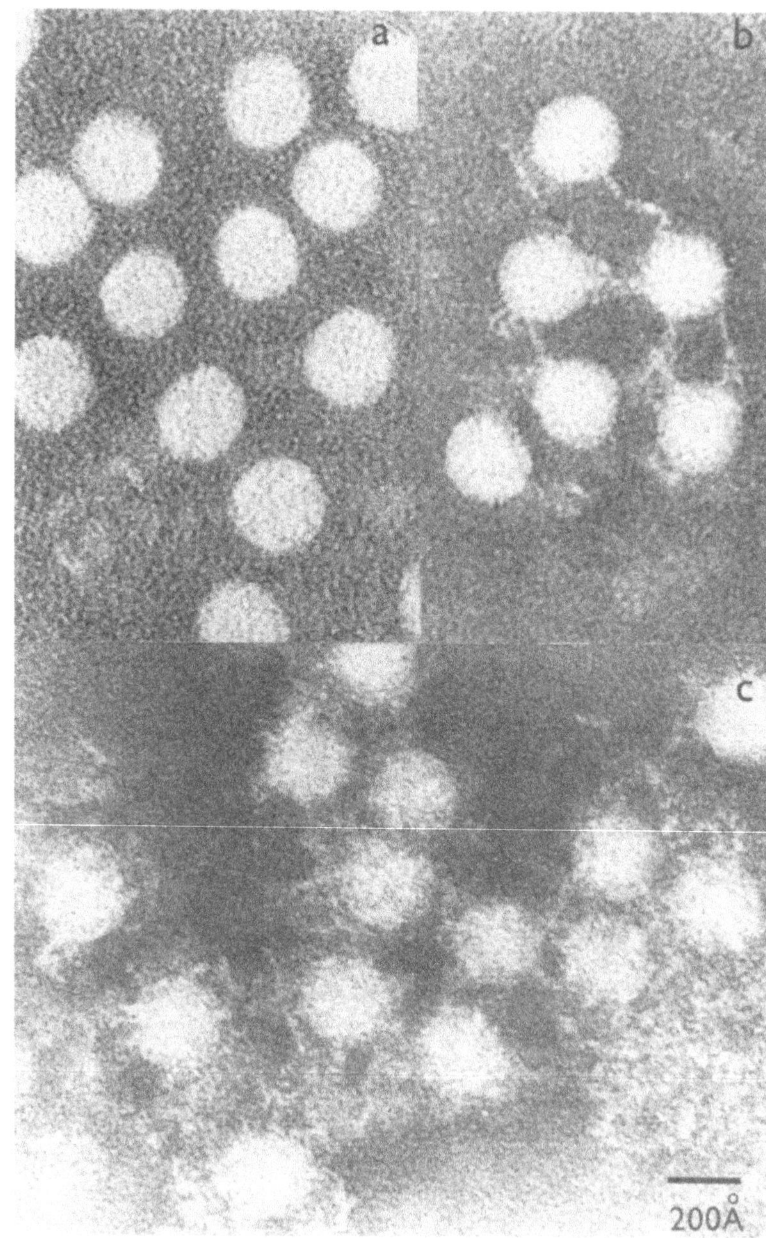

Fig. 2 Electron micrographs of foot-and-mouth disease virus (a) alone; (b) complexed with IgM; (c) complexed with IgG.

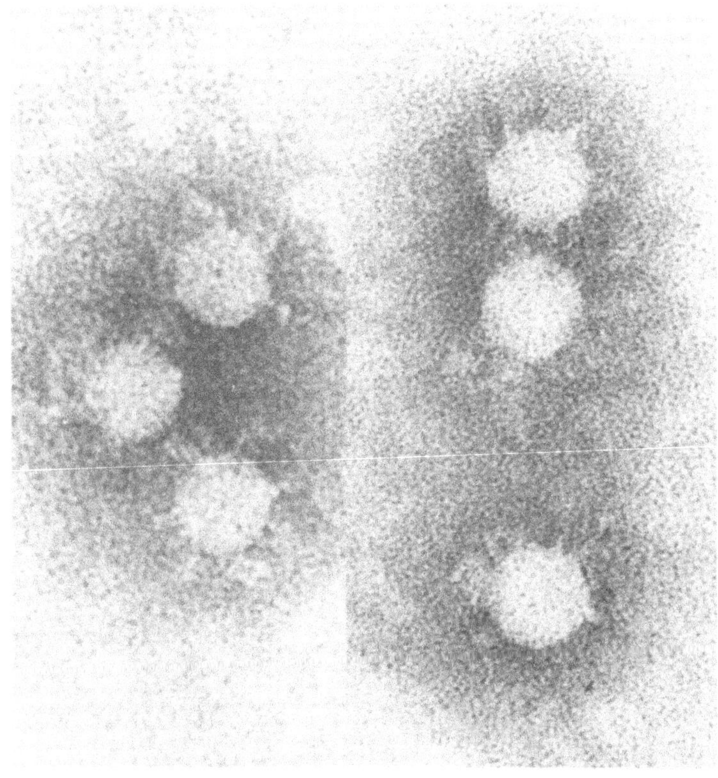

Fig. 3 Electron micrographs of virus complexed with IgG absorbed with the 12S sub-unit.

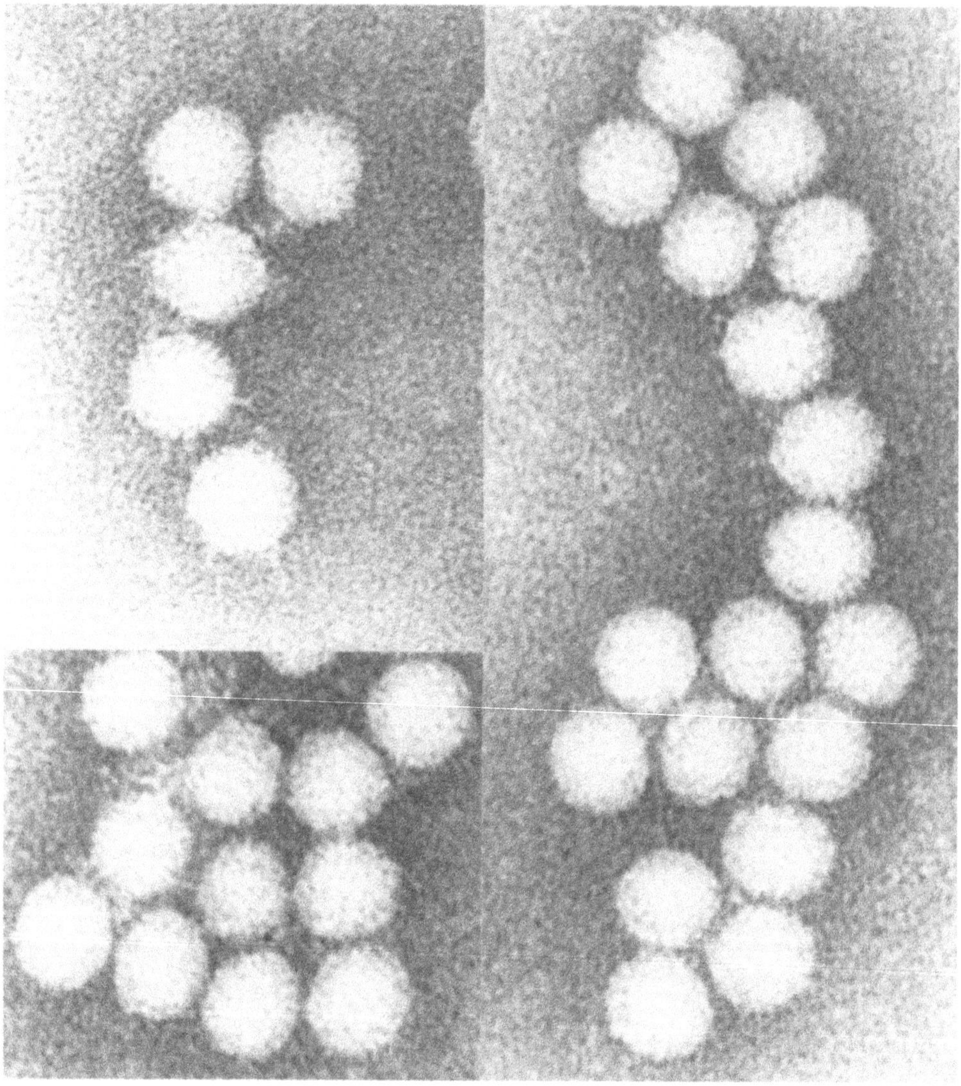

Fig. 4 Electron micrographs of virus complexed with IgG absorbed with trypsin-treated virus particles.

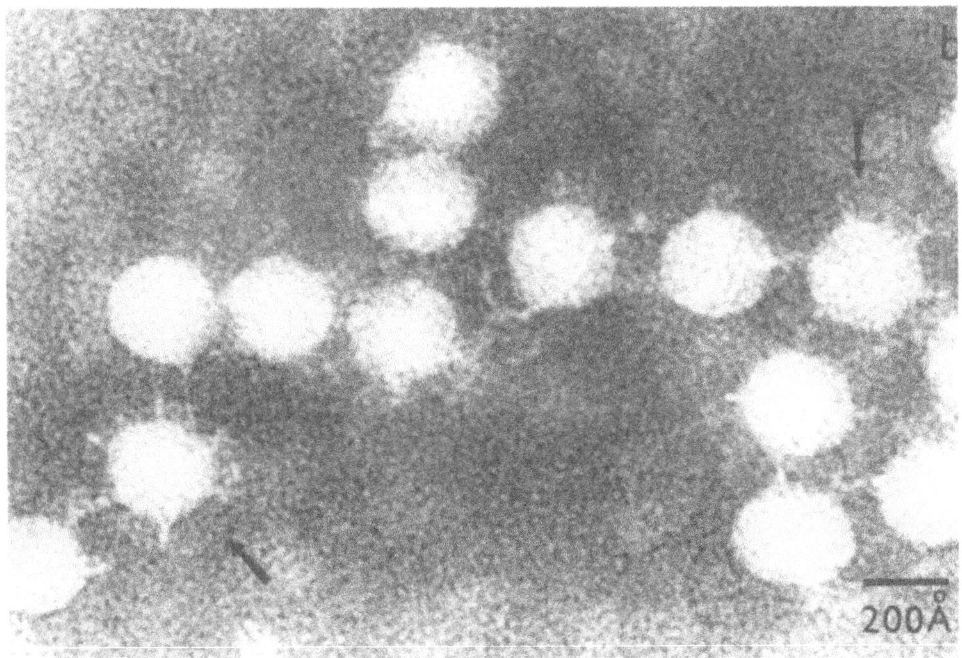

Fig. 5 Electron micrograph of trypsin-treated virus particles complexed with IgG absorbed with the 12S sub-unit. The arrows indicate particles with regularly spaced sites of attachment.

REFERENCES

1. ROWLANDS, D.J., SANGAR, D.V. & BROWN, F. *J. Immunol.*, 1972. (in press).
2. FENWICK, M.L. *Biochem. J.* *107:*851, 1968.
3. NEWMAN, J.F.E. (personal communication).
4. BACHRACH, H.L., TRAUTMAN, R. & BREESE, S.S. *Amer. J. Vet. Res.* *25:*333, 1964.
5. TALBOT, P. & BROWN, F. *J. Gen. Virol.* 1972 (in press).
6. BURROUGHS, J.N., ROWLANDS, D.J., SANGAR, D.V., TALBOT, P. & BROWN, F. *J. Gen. Virol.* *13:*73, 1971.

7. STROHMAIER, K. *Proceedings of 2nd International Congress for Virology*, Budapest, 1971.
8. LIEBERMANN, H. & SCHULZE, P. *Archiv für Experimentelle Veterinärmedizin* *25:*171, 1971.
9. GRAVES, J.H., COWAN, K.M. & TRAUTMAN, R. *Virology* *34:*269, 1968.
10. ROWLANDS, D.J., SANGAR, D.V. & BROWN, F. Unpublished data.
11. BROWN, F. & SMALE, C.J. *J. of Gen. Virol.* *7:*115, 1970.
12. ROWLANDS, D.J., SANGAR, D.V. & BROWN, F. *J. Gen. Virol.* *13:* 85, 1971.

THE ORIGIN OF PANDEMIC STRAINS OF INFLUENZA. EVIDENCE FROM STUDIES OF THE STRUCTURE OF THE HEMAGGLUTININ SUBUNITS

W. G. Laver

Department of Microbiology, The John Curtin School of Medical Research, Australian National University Canberra, Australia

INTRODUCTION

Influenza continues to be one of the major epidemic diseases of man. Pandemics of influenza A occur at irregular intervals, with intervening outbreaks of reduced severity. Between pandemics the virus slowly changes, undergoing gradual alterations in its surface antigens (immunological, or antigenic drift); but the major epidemics are caused by new virus strains having surface antigens unrelated to those of viruses currently circulating.

SURFACE ANTIGENS AND ANTIGENIC VARIATION

Particles of influenza virus possess at least three distinct surface antigens. Two of these, the hemagglutinin and enzyme neuraminidase, exist on different subunits and are virus-coded proteins while the third antigen is a host-cell antigen composed mostly of carbohydrate and covalently attached to the viral proteins.

The antigenic drift, involving gradual changes in the surface antigens of the virus, is thought to result from the selection in an immune population of mutant virus particles having altered antigenic determinants and which therefore possess a growth advantage in the presence of antibody (1,2,3). It has been shown that antigenic mutants isolated *in vitro* by selection with antibody display changes in the amino acid sequence in the polypeptides of the hemagglutinin subunits (4) and it is likely that antigenic drift in the neuraminidase occurs by the same mechanism. The other kind of antigenic variation (major antigenic shift) involves sudden and complete changes in one or both of the surface antigens so that "new" viruses arise to which the population has little or no immunity; it is these viruses which are the cause of the major pandemics of influenza. The origin of the "new" viruses is, however, not known.

EVOLUTION OF A_2 INFLUENZA VIRUSES AND CHARACTERISTICS OF THE HONG KONG STRAIN

The human A_2 influenza viruses offer a natural system for studying the molecular aspects of antigenic variation. The A_2/Asian strain of influenza appeared in man in 1957. This virus possessed hemagglutinin and neuraminidase subunits which were completely unrelated, immunologically, to the hemagglutinin and neuraminidase of the preceding A_0 and A_1 influenza strains. Between 1957 and 1968 antigenic drift occurred in both the hemagglutinin and neuraminidase subunits of A_2/Asian influenza virus and then, in July, 1968, a "new" virus appeared in Southeastern China. This virus (A_2/Hong Kong) caused a very large epidemic in Hong Kong and subsequently spread throughout the rest of the world, replacing the A_2/Asian strains completely. Particles of Hong Kong influenza virus were found to have neuraminidase subunits which were immunologically identical to those of the A_2/Asian strains while the hemagglutinin of Hong Kong influenza and the A_2/Asian strains appeared to be different.

Reports on the extent of this difference, however, varied greatly. Thus, Fazekas (5,6) described hemagglutination-inhibition tests which suggested that considerable similarities existed between the A_2/Asian strains and the Hong Kong strains and this led to the concept of "bridging" strains between these two groups of viruses. Similarly, Dowdle *et al* (7), who used intact viruses both for the preparation of antisera and as test antigens in hemagglutination-inhibition tests, were not able to show a sharp demarcation between the hemagglutinin antigens of the A_2/Asian viruses and the "new" Hong Kong strains.

On the other hand, Schulman and Kilbourne (8), using recombinant viruses (antigenic hybrids), were able to demonstrate that the cross reactions found in hemagglutination-inhibition tests between the A_2/Asian viruses and the "new" Hong Kong strains were spurious, due to antibody against the neuraminidase which was a common antigen to the two groups of viruses.

In the present work we have shown that there was absolutely no serological relationship between the hemagglutinin subunits of Hong Kong influenza and the A_2/Asian strains (although the neuraminidase subunits of the two groups of viruses were related) and we have tried to answer the question, "from where did the hemagglutinin subunits of Hong Kong influenza come?"

Speculation on the Origin of the Hemagglutinin Subunits of Hong Kong Influenza

There seemed to be two possible origins for the "new" hemagglutinin subunits: either they were derived by mutation from those of a preexisting human influenza virus, or they came from some other source such as an animal or avian influenza virus. Although the hemagglutinin subunits of Hong Kong influenza and the A_2/Asian strains were completely different, immunologically, we nevertheless thought that the former could have been derived from the latter by mutation. Relatively few changes in amino acid sequence could have caused the polypeptides of the hemagglutinin subunits to refold in such a way as to expose completely new antigenic determinants. In this case, however, the amino acid sequences of the "old" and "new" hemagglutinin subunits would not be vastly different.

On the other hand, if the "new" hemagglutinin subunits were derived (for instance by genetic recombination) from an animal or avian influenza virus, there might well be great differences in amino acid sequence between the "old" and the "new" hemagglutinin subunits.

Structure of the Hemagglutinin Subunits

The hemagglutinin subunits of influenza virus shown in Fig. 1 are rod-shaped structures, about 140 Å long and 40 Å wide, with a molecular weight of approximately 150,000 (9). They are composed of two heavy polypeptide chains (of about 60,000 mol. wt.) and two light chains (of about 20,000 mol. wt.) (10). In the intact subunits, the light chain is joined to the heavy chain by -S-S- bond(s) to form a dimer of 80,000 mol. wt. (Fig. 2) and each hemagglutinin subunit contains two of these dimers. The two chains can be separated by SDS- polyacrylamide gel electrophoresis in the presence of dithiothreitol or, on a preparative scale, by sedimentation through a guanidine hydrochloride-dithiothreitol density gradient. Peptide mapping experiments showed that the two chains have quite different amino acid sequences.

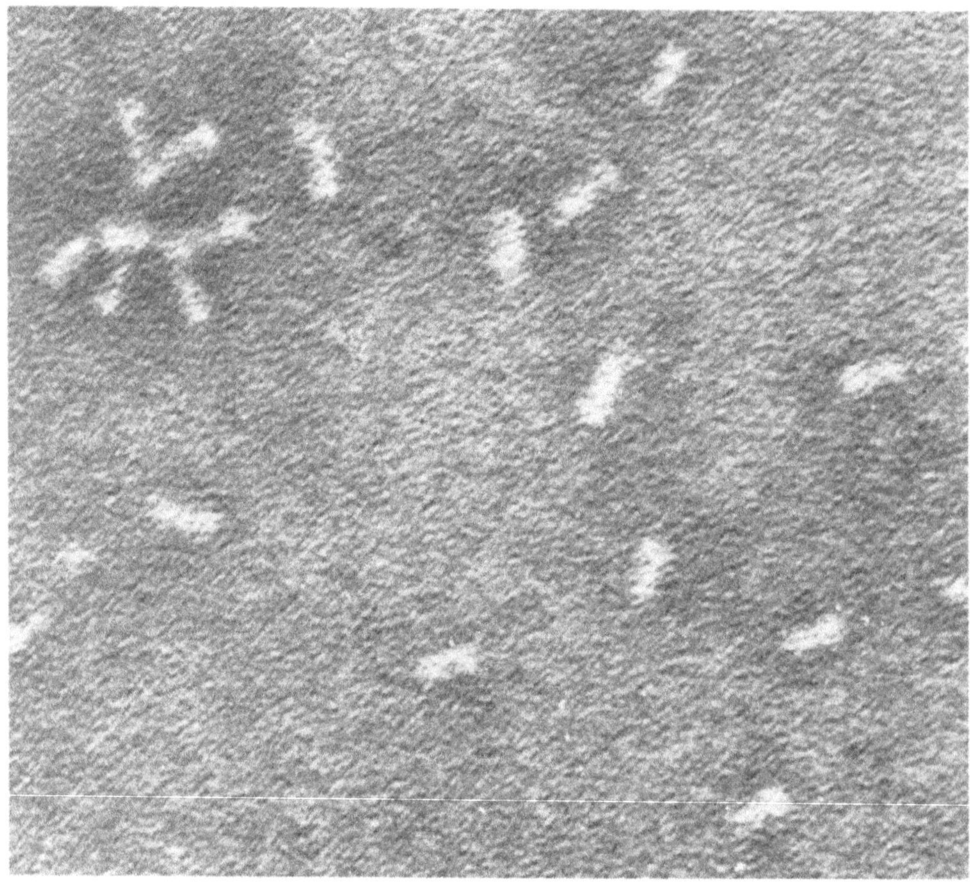

Fig. 1 Electron micrograph of the isolated hemagglutinin subunits of influenza virus in the presence of SDS. The subunits were isolated from a recombinant virus (having A_2/Hong Kong/1968 hemagglutinin and A_0/BEL neuraminidase) by electrophoresis on cellulose acetate strips after disruption of the virus particles with SDS at 20°. These subunits do not hemagglutinate in the presence of SDS; they are "monovalent", attaching to red cells without bridging them. The preparation did, however, have some hemagglutinin activity. It is thought that this was due to a small number of aggregated subunits, some of which can be seen in the electron micrograph. 600,000 X.

Electron micrograph by Nick Wrigley.

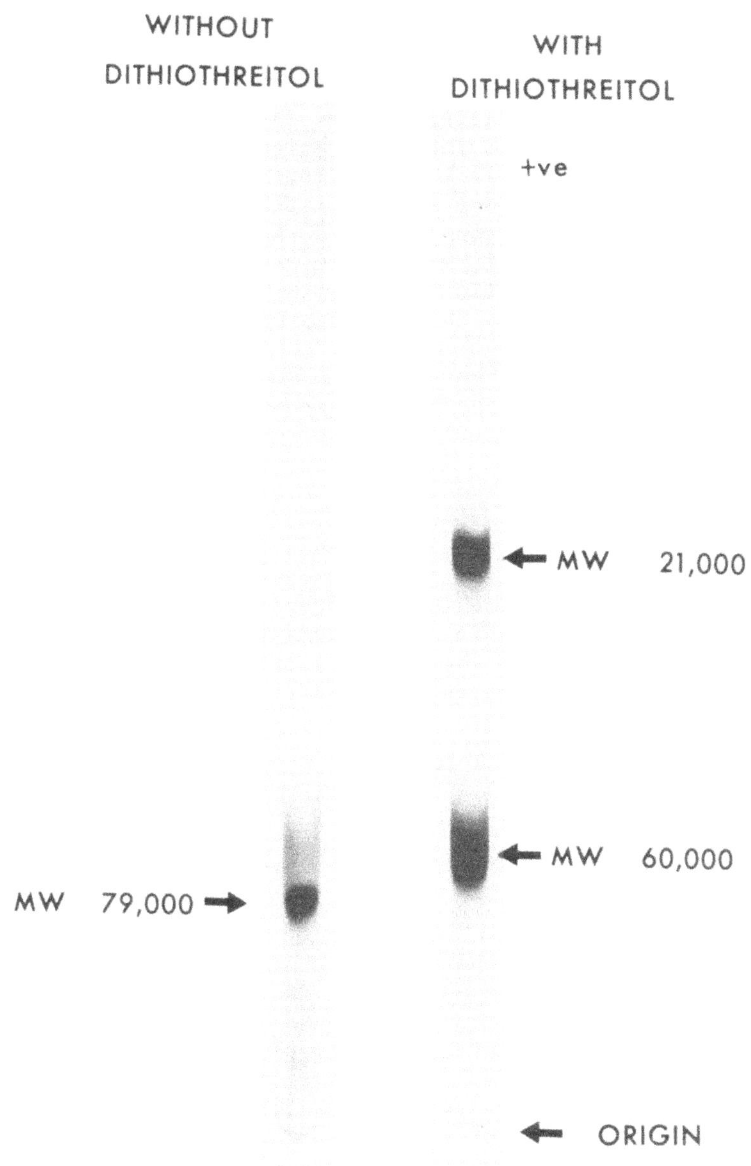

BEL VIRUS HEMAGGLUTININ

Fig. 2 Stained gels showing SDS-polyacrylamide electrophoresis of the hemagglutinin subunits of BEL influenza virus in the presence and absence of dithiothreitol.

Isolation of Hemagglutinin Subunits from A_2 Influenza Viruses

We selected three A_2/Asian strains (A_2/Korea/426/68, A_2/Nederlands/84/68, A_2/Berkeley/1/68) which were isolated in different parts of the world in 1968 before the Hong Kong strain appeared, and three Hong Kong strains isolated between 1968 and 1971 (A_2/Aichi/2/68, A_2/Queensland/7/70, A_2/Memphis/1/71). Antisera prepared against the A_2/Asian viruses cross-reacted strongly in hemagglutination-inhibition tests with the Hong Kong strains (Table 1) in agreement with the findings of others mentioned above.

We then isolated the hemagglutinin subunits from the three A_2/Asian strains and from the three A_2/Hong Kong viruses in the following way. The hemagglutinin subunits of the A_2 viruses were first segregated from the A_2 neuraminidase subunits on to recombinant viruses (antigenic hybrids) containing neuraminidase subunits from an A_0 influenza virus (strain BEL). Disruption of the hybrid viruses with SDS denatured the neuraminidase and internal proteins and the A_2 hemagglutinin subunits could then be isolated in pure form by electrophoresis in buffer containing SDS (Fig. 3). Separation of the hemagglutinin and neuraminidase subunits of the parental A_2 virus could not be done directly in this way, since both were stable in the presence of SDS.

RESULTS

Hemagglutinin Subunits of A_2/Asian Influenza Viruses Not Related Immunologically to Those of the Hong Kong Strain

Antisera prepared to the hemagglutinin subunits isolated from virus grown in chicken embryos contained extremely high levels of antibody to the hemagglutinin antigen and low levels of antibodies to the carbohydrate host antigen covalently attached to the subunits, but did not react with any of the other virus-coded structural antigens. These sera were used in hemagglutination-inhibition tests with the A_2 viruses grown in duck embryos, thus avoiding the problem of steric inhibition of hemagglutination by antibodies to the neuraminidase and host antigens obtained when intact viruses were used. The result of these tests showed that there was no serological relationship between the hemagglutinin antigens of the A_2/Asian and the "new" Hong Kong strains of influenza A_2 viruses (Table 2). It was also noticed that considerable antigenic variation in the hemagglutinin occurred in the A_2/Asian influenza strains isolated in 1968 before Hong Kong influenza appeared, whereas little or no variation was found in the three Hong Kong strains isolated over a three year period.

TABLE I

CROSS-REACTIONS IN HEMAGGLUTININ-INHIBITION TESTS BETWEEN A_2 VIRUSES USING ANTISERA TO WHOLE VIRUS PARTICLES

Antisera to Intact Viruses	HI Titers Against Intact Viruses				
	A_2/Asian Strains			Hong Kong Strains	
	A_2/Korea/68	A_2/Ned/68	A_2/Berk/68	A_2/Aichi/68	A_2/Qld/70
A_2/Korea/68	3,900	1,200	1,100	250	150
A_2/Ned/68	1,200	10,000	4,100	790	650
A_2Berk/68	4,500	2,400	8,300	560	320
A_2/Aichi/68	1,180	370	650	6,500	5,100
A_2/Qld/70	2,900	740	790	8,900	6,700

All viruses were grown in chicken embryos.

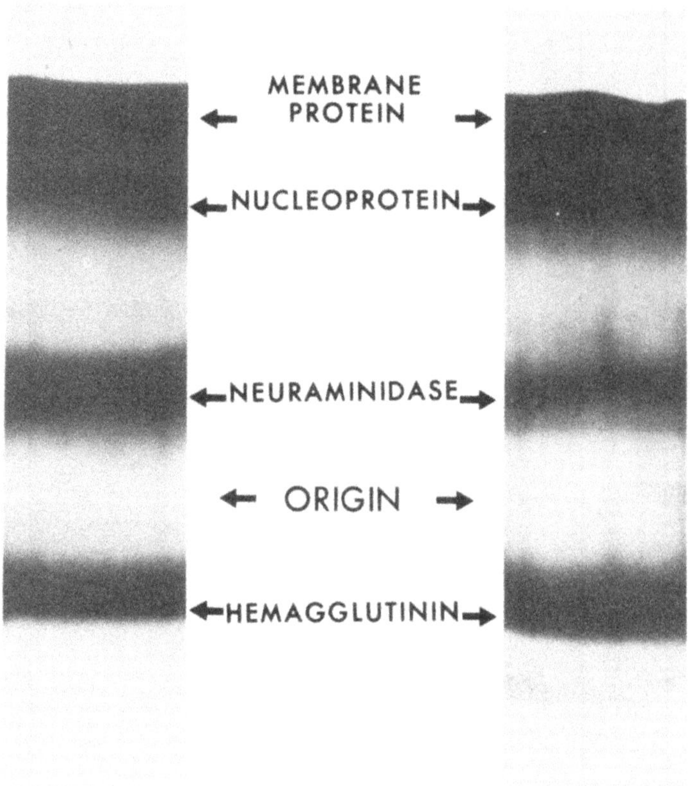

Fig. 3 Cellulose acetate strips, stained with Coomassie Blue, showing the electrophoretic separation of the proteins of two of the recombinant viruses, one (A_2/Korea/426/68$^{(HA)}$-A_0/Bel$^{(NA)}$) having A_2/Asian hemagglutinin subunits and the other (A_2/Memphis/1/71$^{(HA)}$ - A_0/Bel$^{(NA)}$) having the hemagglutinin subunits of one of the Hong Kong strains. The virus particles were disrupted with cold (20°) SDS and the proteins separated by electrophoresis on cellulose acetate strips as previously described (15). The bands containing the biologically active hemagglutinin subunits were eluted from companion (unstained) strips. The proteins in the other bands have been identified as the neuraminidase, ribonucleoprotein and internal (or membrane) protein from their mobilities during polyacrylamide gel electrophoresis (10, 16, 17).

TABLE II

CROSS-REACTIONS IN HEMAGGLUTINATION-INHIBITION TESTS BETWEEN A_2 VIRUSES USING ANTISERA TO ISOLATED HEMAGGLUTININ SUBUNITS FROM VIRUSES GROWN IN A DIFFERENT HOST

Antisera to Hemagglutinin Subunits Isolated from Viruses Grown in Chicken Embryos	HI Titers Against Intact Viruses Grown in Duck Embryos					
	A_2/Asian Strains			Hong Kong Strains		
	A_2/Korea/68	A_2/Ned/68	A_2Berk/68	A_2/Aichi/68	A_2/Qld/70	A_2/Memphis/71
A_2/Korea/68	35,000	1,400	17,000	<20	<20	<20
A_2/Ned/68	2,900	89,000	8,900	<20	<20	<20
A_2/Berk/68	2,200	2,400	8,300	<20	<20	<20
A_2/Aichi/68	<20	<20	<20	38,000	35,000	18,000
A_2/Qld/70	<20	<20	<20	48,000	31,000	11,000
A_2/Memphis/71	<20	<20	<20	9,400	9,400	9,200

Peptide Maps of the Light and Heavy Polypeptide Chains from A_2/Asian and "New" Hong Kong Hemagglutinin Subunits

The hemagglutinin subunits were dissociated by treatment with guanidine hydrochloride and dithiothreitol and the light and heavy polypeptide chains were separated by centrifugation on guanidine hydrochloride-dithiothreitol density gradients as previously described (10). Each of the isolated polypeptide chains was then digested with trypsin and the tryptic peptides were mapped.

Maps of the tryptic peptides from the light chains of the hemagglutinin subunits from the six A_2 influenza viruses are shown in Fig. 4 (a and b). The maps of the light chains from the three A_2/Asian strains isolated in 1968, before Hong Kong virus appeared, (Fig. 4a) differ from one another in a few peptides, but all are obviously related and it is immediately obvious that none bear any resemblance to the maps of the light chains from the three Hong Kong strains (Fig. 4b), all of which appear to be the same. These maps were completely reproducible, and duplicate maps were identical, even in the most faintly staining peptides.

Maps of the tryptic peptides from the heavy chains of the hemagglutinin subunits of the six A_2 viruses are shown in Fig. 5 (a and b). The results were similar to those obtained with the light chains. Thus, the maps of the heavy chains from the three Hong Kong strains (Fig. 5b) are completely different from the maps of the heavy chains from the A_2/Asian viruses (Fig. 5a).

The maps of the heavy chains from each of the three Hong Kong strains were identical with one or two clear-cut exceptions. The most noticeable difference was a peptide present on the A_2/Aichi/68 and A_2/Memphis/71 maps which had shifted to a much lower position on the A_2/Queensland/70 map. Amino acid analysis of these peptides showed that the peptides from A_2/Aichi/68 and A_2/Memphis/71 contained a leucine residue which was replaced by a glutamine residue in A_2/Queensland/70. As well as this difference, two peptides near the origin of the A_2/Aichi/68 map were missing from the map of the A_2/Memphis/71 strain (Fig. 5b). The maps of the heavy chains from the hemagglutinin subunits of the A_2/Asian viruses showed that many differences existed between the three strains. Nevertheless, these latter maps were all obviously related.

None of the maps showed any resemblance to the maps of the light and heavy chains of the hemagglutinin subunits of A_0/BEL influenza virus, the parental virus which donated the neuraminidase subunits to the recombinant viruses from which the A_2 hemagglutinin subunits were isolated.

<u>Figs. 4a and 4b</u> (on following pages)

Maps of the tryptic peptides (soluble at pH 6.5) from the light polypeptide chains of the hemagglutinin subunits:

(4a) three strains of A_2/Asian influenza isolated in 1968 before the occurrence of the Hong Kong influenza pandemic;

(4b) three strains of Hong Kong influenza isolated in different parts of the world in 1968, 1970 and 1971. Electrophoresis at pH 6.5 was followed by ascending chromatography in pyridine-isoamyl alcohol-water (35:35:30). Peptides were stained with ninhydrin. The spots around the periphery of the maps are reference substances. Glycine, histidine and arginine were used as markers of electrophoretic mobility; a mixture of these amino acids was applied at the top of the map and electrophoresed in parallel with the tryptic peptides. Following electrophoresis, a mixture of leucine and phenol red was applied at each side of the map and these markers were chromatographed together with the peptides. The positions of the various reference substances and the position of the phenol red marker added to the tryptic peptides before mapping are shown. Arrows indicate obvious differences between peptide maps.

ARGININE
HISTIDINE
GLYCINE
PHENOL RED
A2/NED/68
LIGHT CHAIN
LEUCINE
LEUCINE
A2/BERKELY/68
LIGHT CHAIN
A2/KOREA/68
LIGHT CHAIN
CHROMATOGRAPHY
ORIGIN
— ve
+ ve
ELECTROPHORESIS

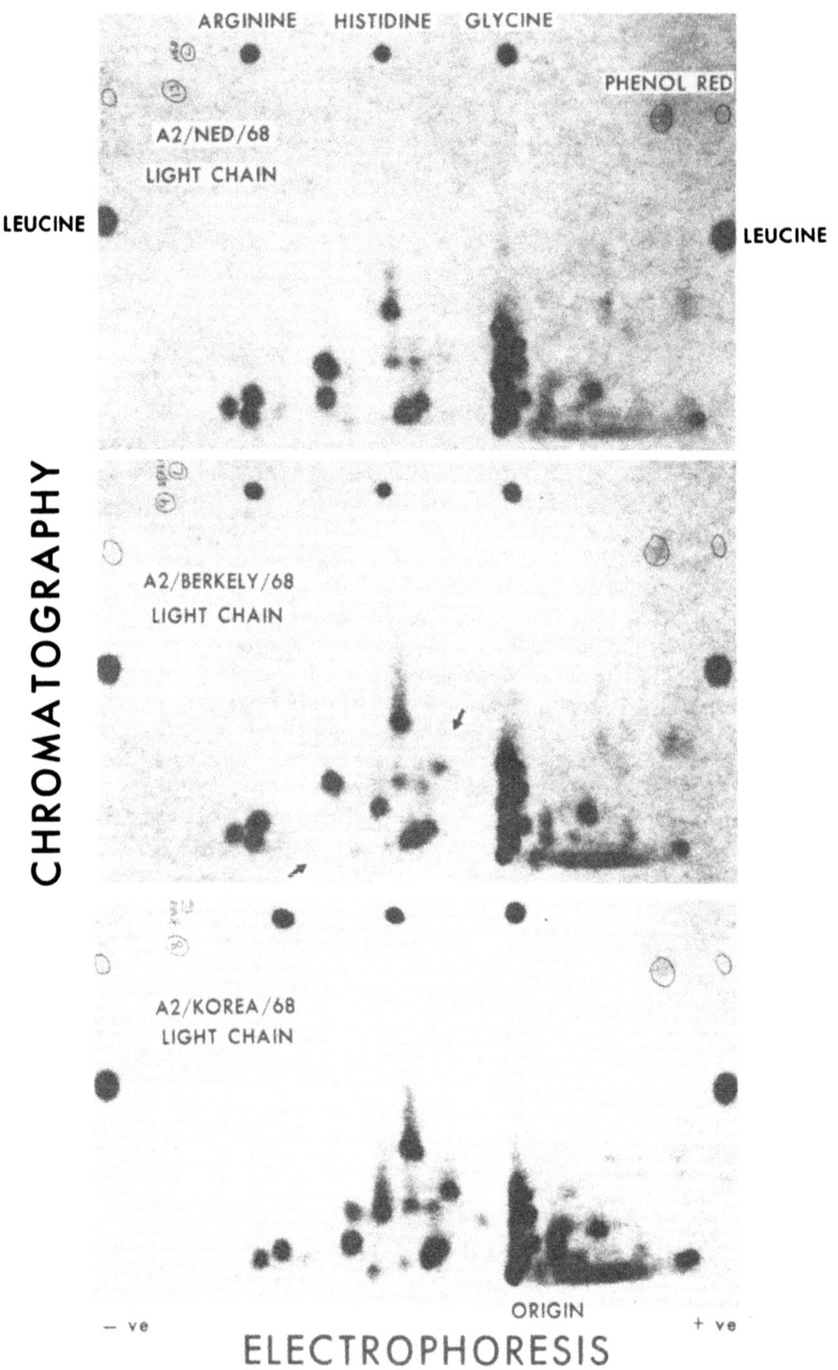

Fig. 4a

ARGININE
HISTIDINE
GLYCINE
PHENOL RED
A2/MEMPHIS/71
LIGHT CHAIN
LEUCINE
LEUCINE
A2/AICHI/68
LIGHT CHAIN
A2/QLD/70
LIGHT CHAIN
CHROMATOGRAPHY
— ve
ORIGIN
+ ve
ELECTROPHORESIS

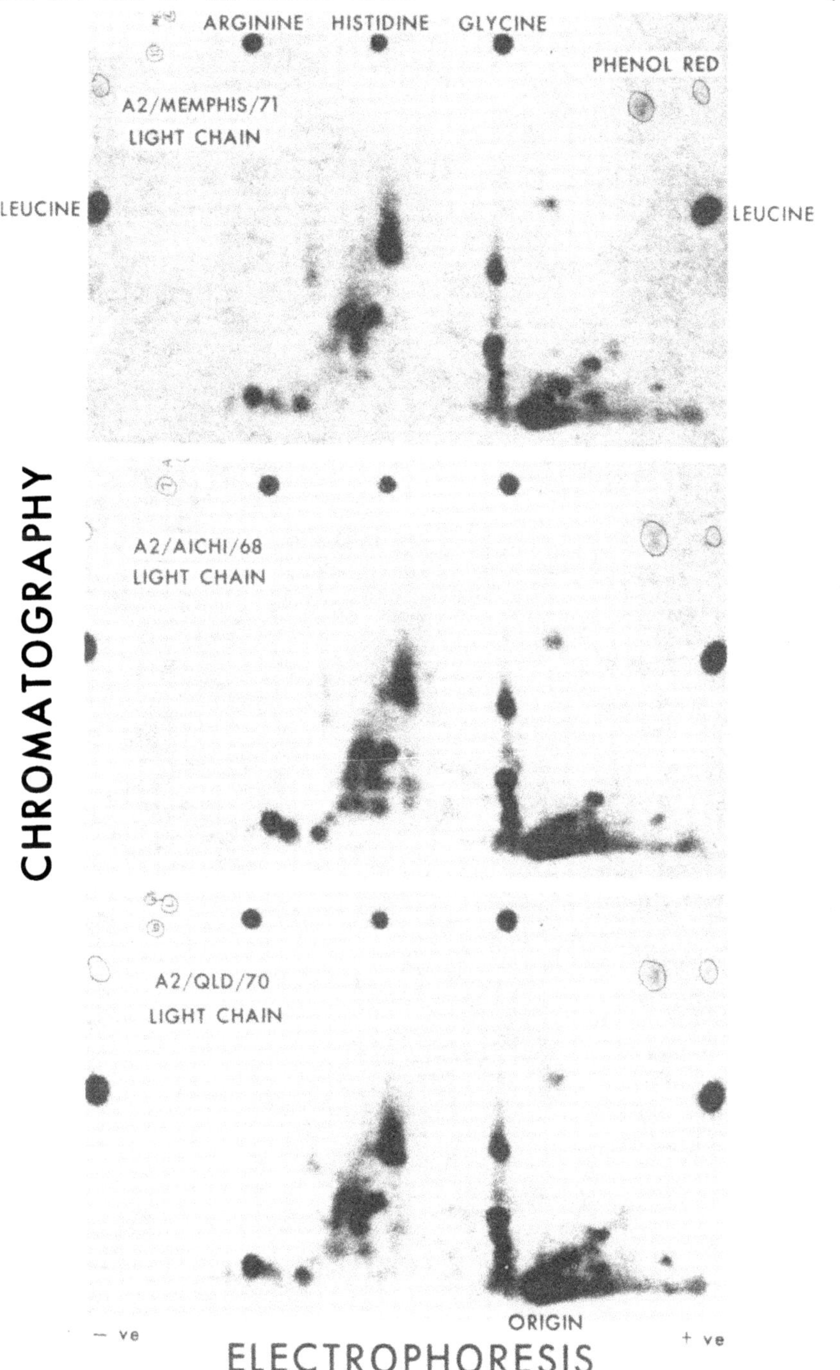

Fig. 4b

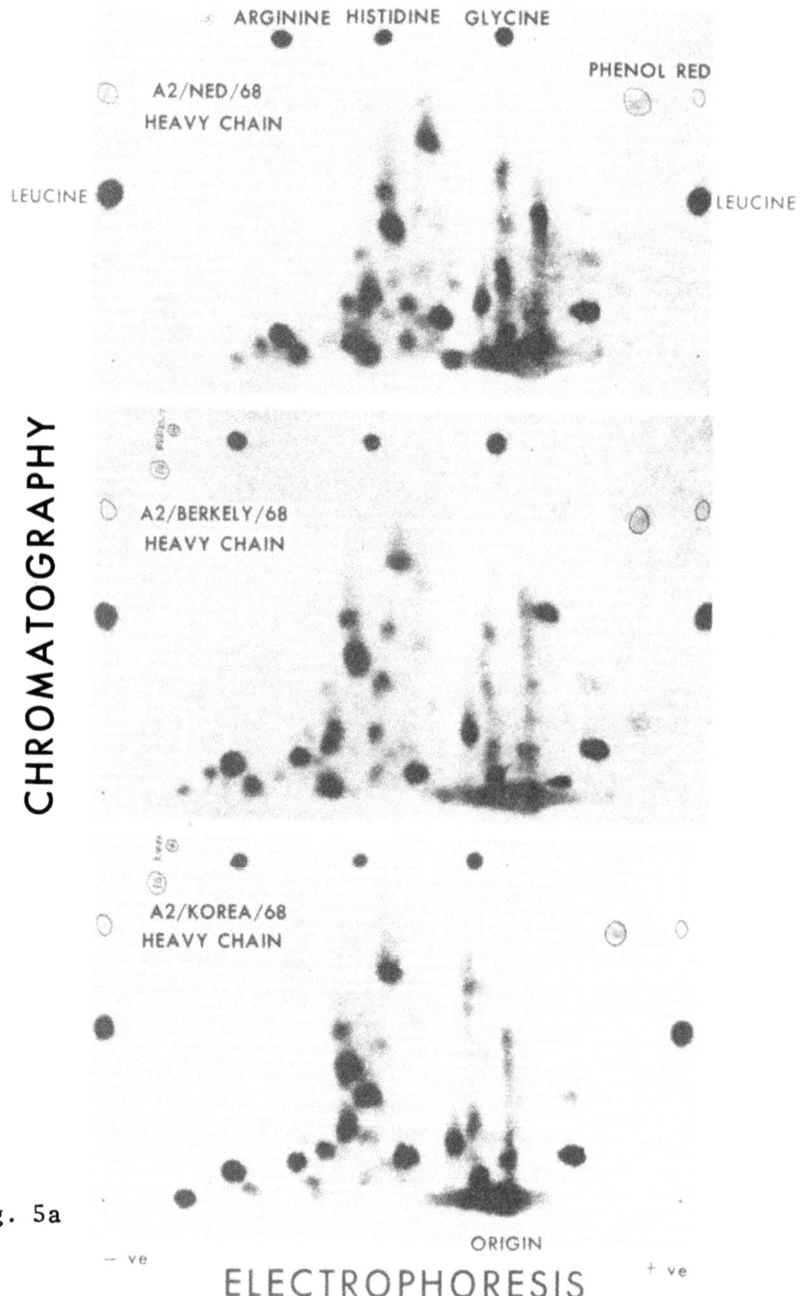

Fig. 5a

Figs. 5a and 5b: Maps of the tryptic peptides from the heavy polypeptide chains of the hemagglutinin subunits. Virus strains and mapping procedure used are as described in Figs. 4a and 4b.

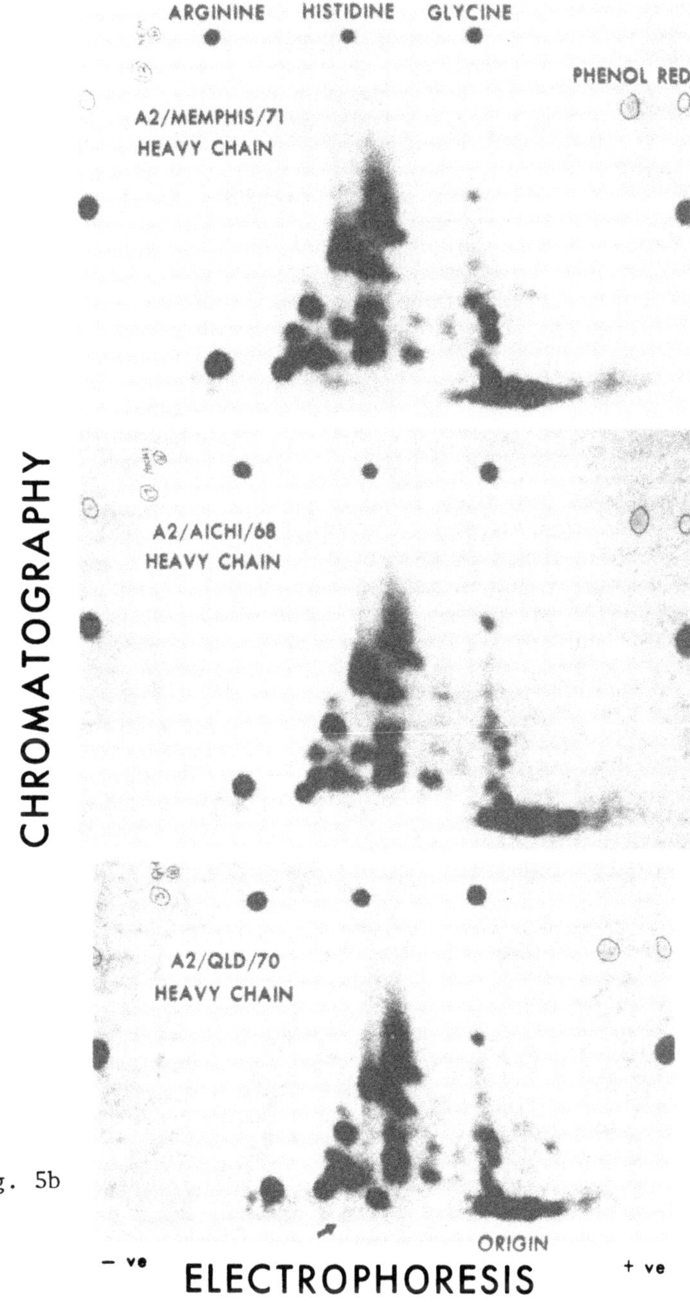

Fig. 5b

Figs. 5a and 5b: Arrows indicate peptides eluted from the maps and analyzed for amino acids.

CONCLUSIONS

Origin of the Hemagglutinin Subunits of Hong Kong Influenza

The findings that the "new" Hong Kong hemagglutinin subunits contained polypeptide chains which differ greatly in amino acid sequence from those of the A_2/Asian viruses suggest that Hong Kong virus may not have come about by mutation from a preexisting human influenza virus. Alternatively, it is proposed that it may have arisen by the selection in a partially immune population of a genetic recombinant. It is also possible that Hong Kong influenza arose as the result of a mutation in an animal or avian virus, giving a virus with the capacity to infect and spread in man. However, particles of Hong Kong influenza have neuraminidase subunits which are immunologically identical to those of the A_2/Asian human influenza viruses and this lends support to the suggestion that Hong Kong influenza arose by recombination rather than by mutation. Genetic recombination between animal, avian, and human influenza viruses has been obtained in the laboratory (11-13) and *in vivo* (14) and there is no reason to suppose that genetic interactions between human and animal or avian influenza viruses do not occur in nature.

It is postulated that Hong Kong influenza virus is a recombinant which was formed as the result of the mixed infection of a susceptible host with an animal or avian influenza virus and a human A_2/Asian virus. The animal (or avian) virus could have donated the hemagglutinin subunits of A_2/Hong Kong/1968 virus and the neuraminidase subunits could have come from the human A_2/Asian strain.

SUMMARY

Hemagglutinin subunits were isolated from three strains of A_2/Asian influenza obtained in 1968 before the occurrence of the Hong Kong influenza pandemic, and from three strains of Hong Kong influenza isolated in different parts of the world in 1968, 1970 and 1971. Antisera prepared against the pure hemagglutinin subunits isolated from these viruses grown in chicken embryos were tested in hemagglutination-inhibition tests with the viruses grown in duck embryos, thus eliminating the spurious cross-reactions due to antibodies to the neuraminidase and host antigens found when intact viruses were used. The results of these tests showed that the hemagglutinin subunits of the Hong Kong strains were completely different, immunologically, from those of the A_2/Asian viruses. (The neuraminidase subunits of Hong Kong influenza, on the other hand, have been found to be similar to those of the A_2/Asian strains.)

The hemagglutinin subunits were dissociated by treatment with guanidine hydrochloride and dithiothreitol and the light and heavy polypeptide chains were separated by centrifugation. Each of the isolated polypeptide chains was then digested with trypsin and the tryptic peptides were mapped. The maps showed that the amino acid sequences in the polypeptide chains from the hemagglutinin subunits of the A_2/Asian viruses isolated in 1968 differed greatly from those in the polypeptide chains of the Hong Kong strains. Striking differences occurred in both the light and heavy chains. On the other hand, the maps of the light chains from the three Hong Kong strains were similar to each other, and the maps of the heavy chains were identical, with the exception of one or two peptides only. The maps from the three A_2/Asian 1968 strains differed in a number of peptides (both in the light and heavy chains) but none bore any resemblance to the maps of the Hong Kong strains.

These results suggest that the hemagglutinin subunits of Hong Kong influenza were not derived by mutation from a preexisting human A_2 strain; it is thought that a more reasonable explanation for their origin is that they came, probably by genetic recombination, from an animal or avian influenza virus.

ACKNOWLEDGEMENT

This work was done in collaboration with Dr. R. G. Webster.

REFERENCES

1. FRANCIS, T. JR. & MAASSAB, H.F. Influenza viruses. In: Horsfall and Tamm, Viral and Rickettsial Infections of Man, pp. 689-740, 4th edition, Lippincott, Philadelphia (1965).
2. ARCHETTI, I. & HORSFALL, F.L. JR. *J. Exp. Med.* *92:*441, 1950.
3. HAMRE, D., LOOSLI, C.G. & GERBER, P. *J. Exp. Med.* *107:*829, 1958.
4. LAVER, W.G. & WEBSTER, R.G. *Virology* *34:*193, 1968.
5. FAZEKAS, de ST. GROTH, S. *Bull. World Health Organ.* *41:*651, 1969.
6. FAZEKAS, de ST. GROTH, S. *Arch. Environ. Health* *21:*293, 1970.
7. DOWDLE, W.R., COLEMAN, M.T., HALL, E.C. & KNEZ, V. *Bull. World Health Organ.* *41:*419, 1969.
8. SCHULMAN, J.L. & KILBOURNE, E.D. *Proc. Nat. Acad. Sci. U.S.* *63:*326, 1969.
9. LAVER, W.G. & VALENTINE, R.C. *Virology* *38:*105, 1969.
10. LAVER, W.G. *Virology* *45:*275, 1971.

11. TUMOVA, B. & PEREIRA, H.G. *Virology 27:*253, 1965.
12. EASTERDAY, B., LAVER, W.G., PEREIRA, H.G. & SCHILD, G.C. *J. Gen. Virol. 5:*83, 1969.
13. KILBOURNE, E.D. *Science 160:*74, 1968.
14. WEBSTER, R.G., CAMPBELL, C.H. & GRANOFF, A. *Virology 44:* 317, 1971.
15. LAVER, W.G. *J. Mol. Biol. 9:*109, 1964.
16. COMPANS, R.W., KLENK, H.D., CALIGUIRI, L.A. & CHOPPIN, P.W. *Virology 42:*880, 1970.
17. SCHULZE, I.T. *Virology 42:*890, 1970.

IMMUNOGENIC PROPERTIES OF NATIVE, RECONSTITUTED AND HYBRID MEMBRANES OF MYCOPLASMAS

Shmuel Razin

Hebrew University-Hadassah Medical School

Jerusalem, Israel

The localization in the mycoplasma cell of the antigens responsible for the immunological response of the infected animal is of great interest for the development of vaccines composed of cell fractions rather than whole cells. It seems warranted to assume that, as in other microorganisms, the major immunogens are surface antigens located in the cell mambrane. That this is so is indicated in several recent papers (1-3). Growth and metabolism of the mycoplasmas were inhibited by antisera prepared against the membrane fraction, but not against the cytoplasmic fraction. In most mycoplasmas, membrane proteins appear to be the major immunogens, while in *M. pneumoniae*, the human pathogen, several membrane glycolipids fulfill this function. The serological characterization of membrane lipids is fairly easy compared with the antigenic analysis of membrane proteins, whose solubilization poses special problems. All the procedures known so far, in particular solubilization by detergents, involve variable degrees of protein denaturation. Nevertheless, our results indicate that the immunological activities of membrane proteins resist inactivation by detergents far better than the enzymic activities. The use of deoxycholate for solubilization and fractionation by gel filtration of *Acholeplasma laidlawii* membrane proteins enabled the separation of a fraction highly enriched in antigens which elicit the production of growth and metabolism-inhibiting antibodies. The relative resistance of membrane antigens to inactivation by detergents enabled the recovery of immunogenic activity in reconstituted membranes formed by reaggregation of detergent-solubilized membranes (2). Moreover, in this way hybrid membranes containing membrane antigens of two different mycoplasmas could be formed. Hybrid membranes have recently been shown by us (3,4) to provide an efficient tool in the preparation of specific and potent antisera to several membrane lipids. Purified glycolipids of *M. pneumoniae* and cytolipin H of spleen cells, incapable of eliciting an antibody response by themselves, became highly immunogenic when bound to membrane proteins of *A. laidlawii* by the reconstitution process. Possible applications of the reconstitution technique to the immunological characterization of biomembrane components have been studied.

REFERENCES

1. HOLLINGDALE, M.R. & LEMCKE, R.M. *J. Hyg. (Camb.)* *67*:585, 1969.
2. KAHANE, I. & RAZIN, S. *J. Bacteriol.* *100*:187, 1969.
3. RAZIN, S., PRESCOTT, B. & CHANOCK, R.M. *Proc. Natl. Acad. Sci. U.S.A.* *67*:590, 1970.
4. RAZIN, S., CHANOCK, R.M., GRAF, L. & RAPPORT, M.M. *Proc. Soc. Exp. Biol. Med.* *138*:404, 1971.

THE ANTIBODY RESPONSE TO DIFFERENT MEASLES VIRUS ANTIGENS UNDER VARIOUS CONDITIONS OF IMMUNIZATION

E. Norrby[1], A.A. Salmi[2], B. Vandvik[3], B. Hammarskjöld[1] and M. Panelius[4]

Department of Virology, Karolinska Institutet, School of Medicine, Stockholm, Sweden[1]; Department of Virology[2], Department of Neurology[4], University of Turku, Finland; Research Institute of Immunology, Rikshospitalet, Oslo, Norway[3]

A number of attempts have been made to identify different structural components of measles virus (1-6). Hemagglutinating and nonhemagglutinating products have been isolated, but their relationship to different structural components of the virus has not been fully elucidated.

In this paper we discuss techniques which have been developed for preparing isolated nucleocapsids and small particle hemagglutinin (HA). The isolated antigens have been used for characterizing antibody response under different conditions of immunization. Serum samples were collected from patients at different times after ordinary measles infection and from patients with subacute sclerosing panencephalitis (SSPE) and multiple sclerosis (MS). In addition, samples of cerebrospinal fluid (CSF) were obtained from patients with the latter two diseases. These samples were used to evaluate the possible occurrence of a local production of antibodies against measles virus components within the central nervous system (CNS). Locally produced monoclonal IgG was separated by electrophoresis of brain extracts and concentrated samples of CSF from some cases of SSPE. The relationship between the distribution of antibody activities against different virus components and the presence of different clones of IgG was determined.

The occurrence of antibodies against the measles virus hemolysin (HL), as distinct from antibodies against the hemagglutinin (HA), was demonstrated by our findings in these studies. The relative significance of the hemolysin in inducing the production of antibodies giving protection against the disease is discussed. In this connection some preliminary results will be presented from studies of the effect on the hemolysin activity of certain procedures previously employed for preparing inactivated measles vaccines.

PREPARATION OF PURIFIED NUCLEOCAPSIDS AND ISOLATED HEMAGGLUTININ

The detailed procedures employed for purification of nucleocapsids and small particle HA were recently described (7). Nucleocapsids were isolated from concentrates of infected cells treated with a nonionic detergent, Cutscum. The cell extracts were centrifuged in discontinuous sucrose gradients (Fig. 1).

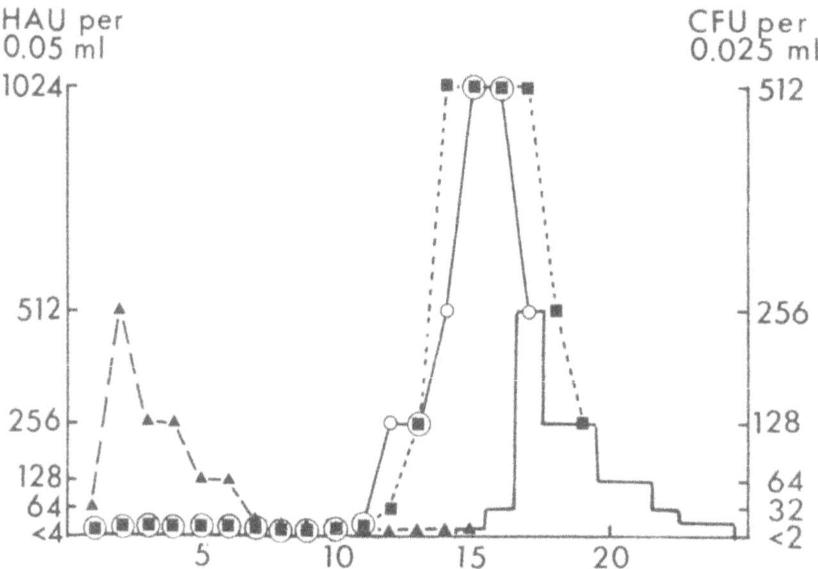

Fig. 1 Distribution of biological activities of cell-associated virus products released by treatment with 1 percent Cutscum (20°C,15') after centrifugation in a discontinuous sucrose gradient (1.5 ml 65 percent, 2 ml 50 percent and 5.5 ml 20 percent sucrose plus 3 ml virus material) at 30,000 rpm (113,000 xg) for 20 h in rotor SW40 (Spinco Div. Beckman Instr. Inc., Calif.). The bottom of the tube is to the left. The following activities were studied: HA (o——o), CF antigen in tests with sera against isolated nucleocapsids (▲--▲) and small particle HA (■-- ■).

Nucleocapsids accumulated at the interphase between the 50 percent and 65 percent sucrose solutions (Fig. 2) and were contaminated with only small amounts of HA which were readily removed by absorption with monkey erythrocytes. The isolated nucleocapsids had properties corresponding to those described for nucleocapsids isolated from other paramyxoviruses. A certain population of nucleocapsids, which was interpreted as representing intact components, sedimented at a rate of 220 to 265 S. By ultrastructural analysis, these nucleocapsids were found to have an average length of 1.15 μm and to represent a helical structure comprising an average of 207 turns (Fig. 2).

Extracellular virus products were used as a source for preparation of purified envelope fragments. Materials were concentrated by forced dialysis and then centrifuged in discontinuous sucrose gradients (Fig. 3). Rapidly sedimenting virus products (intact and slightly damaged virus particles) were recovered from the interphase between the 20 percent and 50 percent sucrose solutions. These products were treated with the nonionic detergent Cutscum and recentrifuged in linear 5 percent to 20 percent sucrose gradients. Under these conditions of centrifugation, nucleocapsids sedimented to the bottom of the tubes. The dominating population of envelope fragments identified by HA and CF tests sedimented at a rate corresponding to 6 and 10 S (Fig. 4). These fragments will be referred to as small particle HA.

THE OCCURRENCE OF CIRCULATING ANTIBODIES AGAINST DIFFERENT MEASLES VIRUS COMPONENTS UNDER VARIOUS CONDITIONS OF IMMUNIZATION

The presence of antibodies against different measles virus antigens was studied in (a) rabbit hyperimmune sera against purified nucleocapsids and small particle HA; (b) acute, early (11 to 40 days after rash) and late (4 to 20 years post infection) convalescent sera from cases of ordinary measles; (c) preparations of ordinary gamma globulin; and (d) serum and CSF samples from patients with SSPE and MS. The following antibody tests were carried out: neutralization (in some cases including the addition of anti-gamma globulin to detect sensitizing antibodies); hemolysis-inhibition (HLI); hemagglutination-inhibition (HI - in most tests antigen treated with Tween 80 and ether (8) was employed, but in certain tests untreated antigen was used); complement-fixation (CF, with extracts of infected cells, purified nucleocapsids and small particle HA as antigens); and immunodiffusion with extracts of infected cells. In immunodiffusion tests two types of antigen preparations were employed. Infected cells extracted with Cutscum were used for the demonstration of antibodies against envelope components and

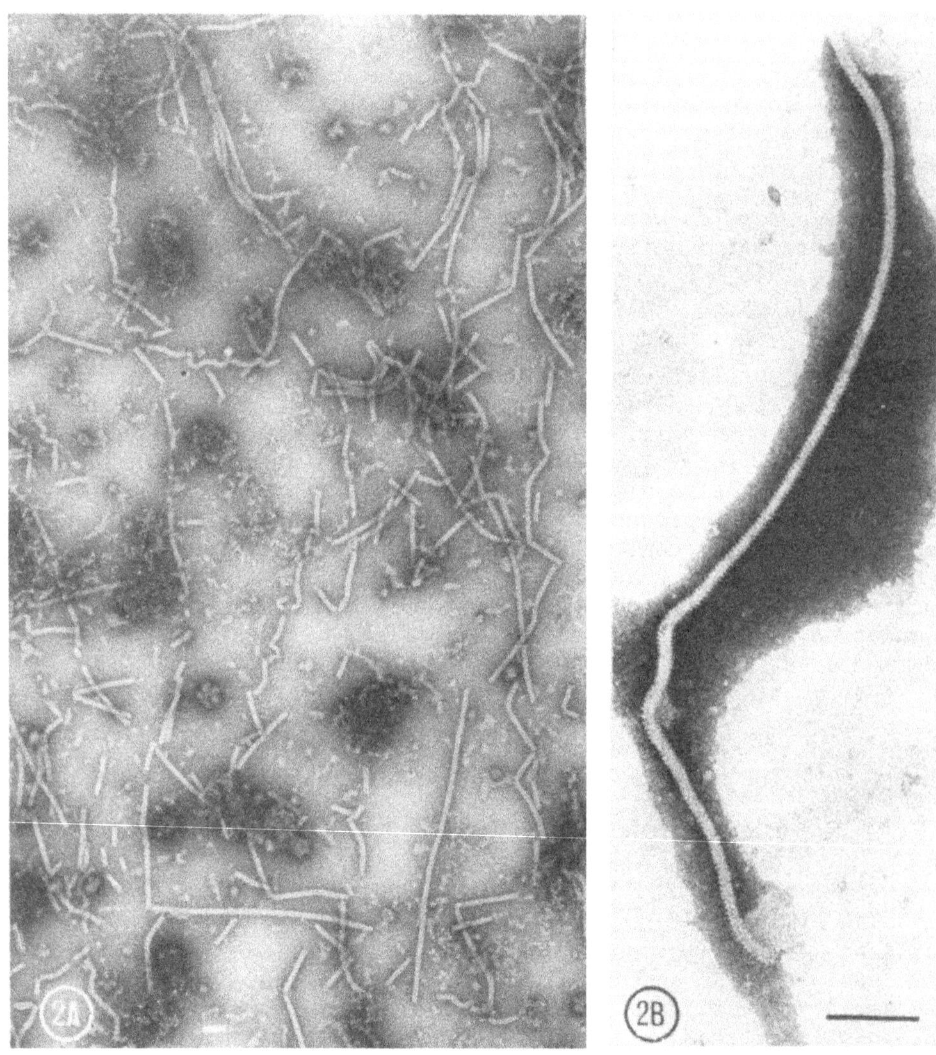

Fig. 2 Ultrastructure of nucleocapsids isolated by centrifugation in a discontinuous sucrose gradient (cf. Fig. 1). The isolated component in figure (B) measures 1.15 μm and comprises 207 helical turns. Negative contrast with STS. Magnification: (A) x 40,000; (B) x 140,000. Bars represent 100 nm.

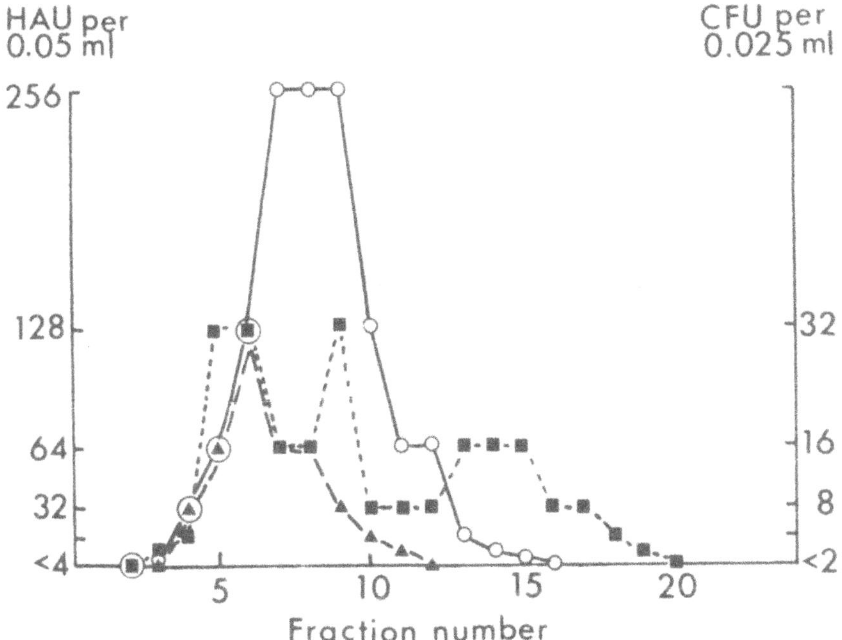

Fig. 3 Distribution of biological activities of concentrated extra-cellular material after centrifugation in a discontinuous sucrose gradient (see Fig. 1) at 30,000 rpm (113,000 xg) for 1.5 h in rotor SW40 (Spinco). The bottom of the tube is to the left. For explanation of symbols see Fig. 1.

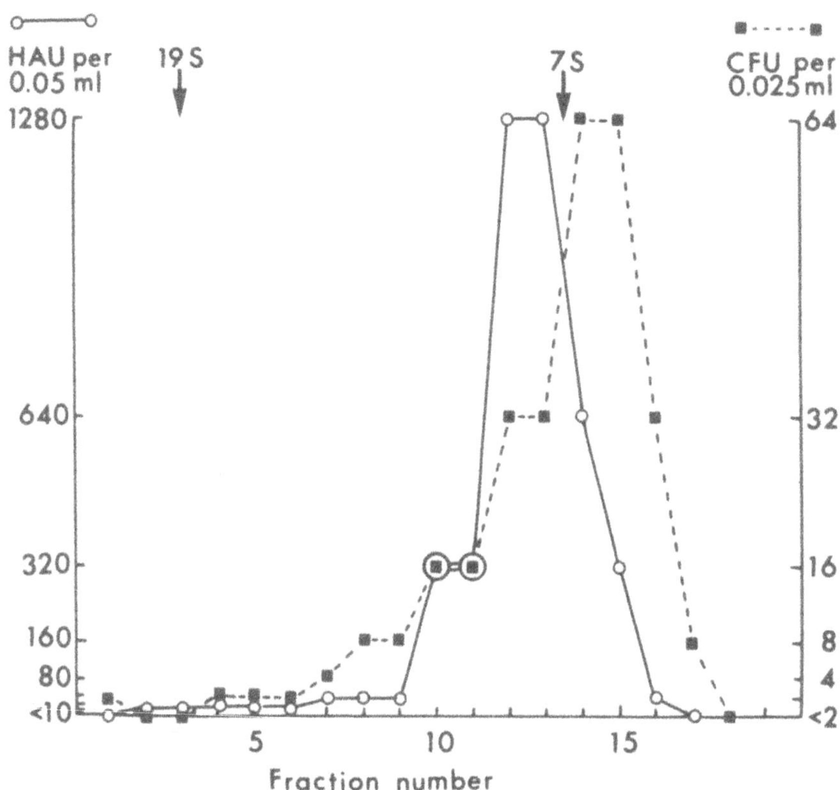

Fig. 4 Distribution of biological activities in a linear 5 percent to 20 percent sucrose gradient after zonal centrifugation at 20,000 rpm (41,000 xg) for 42 h in rotor SW25 (Spinco) of 0.5 percent Cutscum-treated rapidly sedimenting extra-cellular virus products isolated by isopycnic centrifugation in a sucrose gradient (cf Fig. 3). Bottom of tube is to the left. The following activities were determined: HA (o——o), CF antigen in tests with an antiserum against small particle HA (■--■). Nucleocapsid CF antigen was not detectable in any of the fractions.

possibly nonstructural components. For simultaneous identification of antibodies also against nucleocapsid components, the antigen preparations were treated with 0.25 percent sodium dodecylsulphate (SDS). The results obtained were previously summarized for publication (7,9,10).

Rabbit Hyperimmune Sera Against Purified Structural Components

Rabbits were immunized with purified nucleocapsids absorbed with red cells and with small particle HA, prepared as described above. Antisera against nucleocapsids contained antibodies demonstrable only in CF tests with nucleocapsid antigen. In contrast, CF antibodies in antisera against envelope antigen(s) only reacted with small particle HA. These antibodies also were active in neutralization, HLI and HI tests. The specific antibody activities of these hyperimmune sera were further demonstrated in immunodiffusion tests (cf. Fig. 7 and Table 1).

Human Sera and Gamma Globulin

The following principal findings were made:

(a) Early IgG antibodies had a poor neutralizing capacity, presumably due to their low avidity. However, they were capable of sensitizing virions, as demonstrated by the marked increase in their neutralizing activity after addition of anti-gamma globulin.

(b) There was a good correlation between titers of neutralizing and HLI antibodies, as shown in Fig. 5.

(c) The correlation between antibodies demonstrated in HI tests with Tween 80-ether-treated antigen and HLI tests was less strict (Fig. 6).

The presence of HI antibodies always implied a concomitant occurrence of HLI antibodies, but the reverse relationship was not always true. In sera from two patients with MS (J.V., A.V.) and one patient with SSPE, high titers of HLI antibodies were found in the presence of low titers of HI antibodies (Fig. 6, Table 2). In addition, one out of 15 late measles-convalescent sera contained an excess of HLI antibodies.

Possibly HLI antibodies by themselves could give HI if antigen preparations containing HA-associated HL were used instead of Tween 80-ether-treated material.

TABLE I

ANTIBODY ACTIVITIES OF RABBIT HYPERIMMUNE SERA AGAINST NUCLEOCAPSID COMPONENTS AND SMALL PARTICLE HA (Modified from Ref. 7)

Serum Against	Antibody Titers in				
	Neutralization Tests	HLI Tests	HI Tests	CF Tests With	
				Nucleocapsids[a]	Small Particle HA[b]
Nucleocapsid[a] Components	< 2	< 2	< 2	80	< 10
Small Particle[b] HA	5120	2560	4000	< 10	640

(a) Nucleocapsid components used for immunization and, as antigen in CF tests, were prepared by centrifugation of Cutscum-extracted infected cells in discontinuous sucrose gradients (Fig. 1) and subsequent absorbtion with monkey erythrocytes for removal of contaminating HA.

(b) Small particle HA was prepared by zonal centrifugation (Fig. 4) of Cutscum-treated rapidly sedimenting extracellular virus products isolated by centrifugation in discontinuous sucrose gradients (Fig. 3).

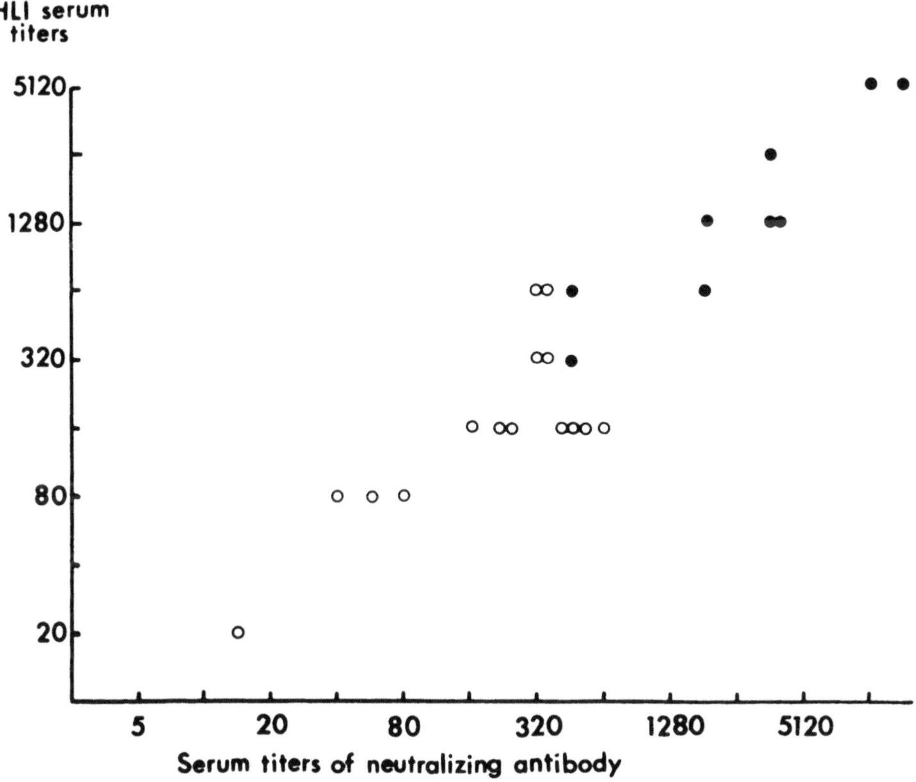

Fig. 5 Correlation between measles virus neutralizing and HLI antibody titers in serum samples from cases of SSPE (•) and MS (o). (From Ref. 10)

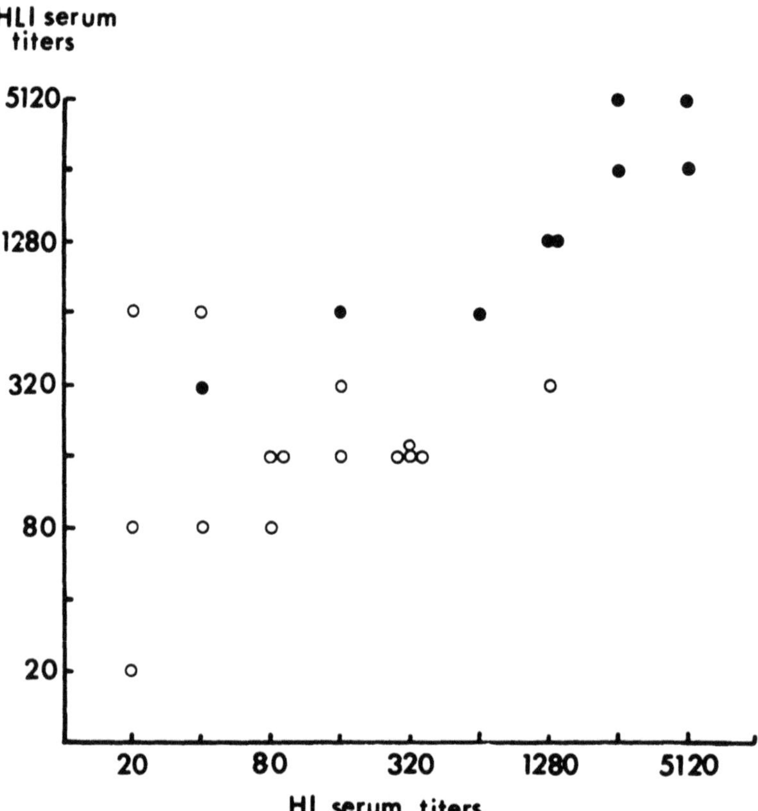

Fig. 6 Correlation between measles virus HI antibody titers with Tween 80-ether-treated antigen and HLI antibody titers in serum samples from cases of SSPE (•) and MS (o).
(From Ref. 10)

TABLE II

HI ANTIBODY TITERS WITH UNTREATED AND TWEEN 80-ETHER-TREATED ANTIGEN AND HLI ANTIBODY TITERS IN HUMAN GAMMA GLOBULIN AND IN LATE CONVALESCENT SERA FROM THREE HEALTHY INDIVIDUALS (GS1, GS4, GS12) AND FROM TWO PATIENTS WITH MULTIPLE SCLEROSIS (J.V., A.V.)
(Modified from Ref. 9)

Serum Sample	HLI Antibody Titer	HI Antibody Titer in Tests with	
		Untreated Antigen	Tween 80-Ether-Treated Antigen
Gamma Globulin	3200	1600	3200
GS4	640	160	320
GS12	1280	160	640
GS1	640	40	20
J.V.	640	80	40
A.V.	640	80	20

In order to investigate this possibility, comparative HI tests were carried out with both treated and untreated antigen preparations (Table 2). As might be expected (8), maximum HI antibody titer of two sera, and of gamma globulin, included as controls, was obtained with Tween 80-ether-treated antigen. In contrast, sera containing an excess of HLI over HI antibodies gave a better inhibition of the HA activity of untreated than of split antigen. It seems likely that the HI activity recorded with untreated antigen in the former case is due to an interaction between antibodies and HA-associated HL.

(d) Among the different measles virus-specific antibodies present both in early and late convalescent sera, antibodies against the nucleocapsid component were quantitatively dominant. This is illustrated by the pattern of immunoprecipitation given by gamma globulin in tests with Cutscum-and SDS-treated antigen preparations (Fig. 7). This pattern of appearance and persistence of antibodies against the measles virus nucleocapsid is different from that of antibodies against the corresponding component of another paramyxovirus, mumps virus. It has been shown (11) that antibodies against the nucleocapsid of mumps virus appear later and disappear more rapidly than antibodies reacting with envelope components.

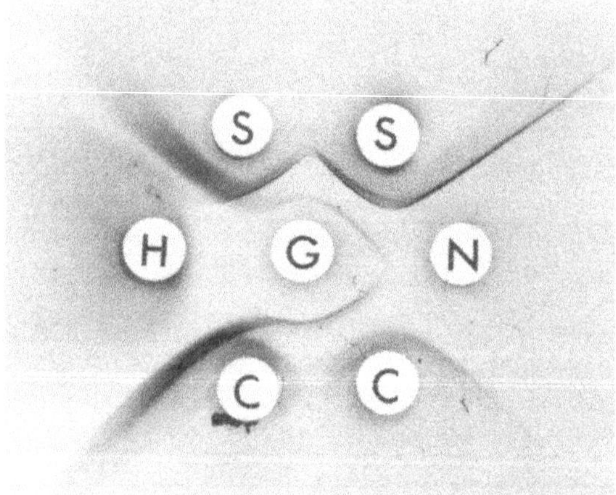

Fig. 7 Characterization of measles virus-specific antibodies in gamma globulin (G) by immunodiffusion. Infected cells extracted with 0.25 percent SDS (S) and 1 percent Cutscum (C) were used and rabbit hyperimmune sera against nucleocapsids (N) and small particle HA (H) were included as references. (From Ref. 9).

In sera from cases of ordinary measles there was a fairly good correlation between the titers of nucleocapsid CF antibodies and HLI antibodies. The latter, as was shown above, represent a good indicator of the overall amount of antibodies present against envelope structures. In sera from patients with SSPE and MS, this correlation was less pronounced (Fig. 8).

Generally, there was a more pronounced diversity of the antibody response to different virus components in samples from cases of SSPE and certain cases of MS than from cases of ordinary measles. Presumably, the condition of what might be described in the former cases as natural hyperimmunization can lead to a preferential antibody response toward one or more of the different virus products. In accordance with previous findings, the titer of circulating measles antibodies was found to be markedly increased in cases of SSPE and moderately increased in some cases of MS.

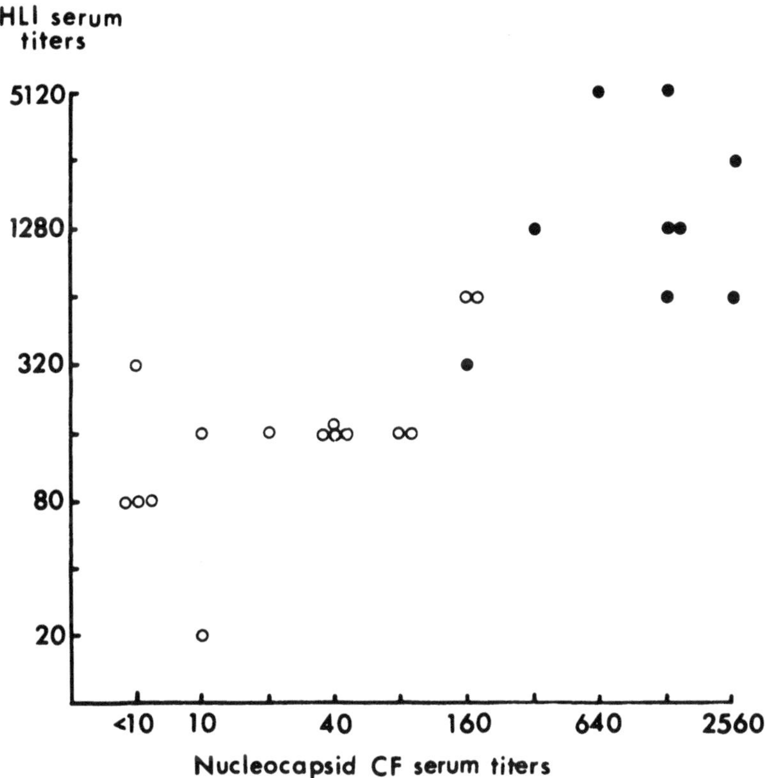

Fig. 8 Correlation between measles virus HLI and nucleocapsid CF serum titers in serum samples from cases of SSPE (•) and MS (o). (From Ref. 10).

A number of neutralization HLI and HI tests, employing two different measles virus strains - Edmonston, and a strain (LEC) derived from a case of SSPE - were carried out using the various types of sera described above. In agreement with previously published data (12), no significant differences in the serological behaviour of the two strains could be detected.

CHARACTERIZATION OF MEASLES VIRUS ANTIBODIES PRODUCED WITHIN THE CNS; ASSOCIATION WITH DIFFERENT CLONES OF IgG

It has been shown previously that the ratio of serum/CSF measles-antibody titers is markedly reduced in patients with SSPE (13). This was concluded from results of simultaneous testing of poliovirus neutralizing and measles virus HI antibodies. The reduced ratio has been considered as implying a local production of measles virus-specific antibodies in the CNS. In the present study, antibodies against the group-specific part of adenovirus vertex capsomers (14) were used as a reference, instead of antibodies against poliovirus. In all eight cases of SSPE studied (four cases included in Table 3) significantly reduced ratios were found in tests for various measles antibodies. Among fifteen cases of MS, eight displayed a reduced ratio of serum/CSF titer in one or more different serological tests for measles virus antibodies. Three out of these eight cases had been chosen for this study because it had been demonstrated previously in preliminary tests that their CSF contained measles virus antibodies, but all other patients were randomly selected from a larger study group of MS patients (15).

Antibodies locally produced in the CNS of patients with SSPE were characterized after electrophoretic separation. Three interlinked questions were asked: (a) Do the different clones of IgG which can be demonstrated by electrophoretic separation of brain extracts or CSF represent antibodies directed against measles virus products or against some other antigens? (b) In the case that the various clones represent measles antibodies, do different clones react with different measles virus antigens? (c) In the case that the antibodies react with different measles virus antigens, does a clone of antibodies which reacts with one special type of antigen preferentially display a particular electrophoretic mobility?

Results obtained so far demonstrate that the answers to questions (a) and (b) and Possibly also (c) are positive. Data to support these conclusions have been summarized in a recent preliminary publication (16).

TABLE III

SERUM/CSF TITER RATIOS OF DIFFERENT MEASLES ANTIBODIES IN SELECTED PATIENTS WITH SSPE AND MS (From Ref. 10)

Patient	Disease	Ratios Between Antibody Titers in Serum and CSF Samples Calculated From:				
		Neutralization Tests	HLI Tests	HI Tests	CF Tests with Extracts of Infected Cells	Adenovirus Penton HE Tests[a]
J.L.	SSPE	10	20	10	25	≥ 80
U.H.	SSPE	40	80	80	50	≥160
L.K.	SSPE	45	20	20	40	320
H.N.	SSPE	13	40	40	25	≥ 80
V.M.	MS	20	20	80	64	512
E.N.	MS	32	20	40	20	≥160
V.K.	MS	23	40	20	32	≥320
S.L.	MS	≥180	40	80	≥80	≥320
J.V.	MS	≥ 90	80	(≥20)[b]	40	≥320
H.S.	MS	90	40	40	16	320
E.K.	MS	≥ 60	≥40	80	10	640
A.V.	MS	≥ 90	80	(≥10)[b]	16	≥ 160

a Determined in tests with adenovirus type 11 penton incomplete HA.

b Low serum titers precluded the calculation of a meaningful ratio.

The correlation found between the occurrence of bands of monoclonal IgG and measles virus-specific antibody activities has been illustrated by results of tests of CSF from one SSPE patient (Fig. 9). The monoclonal nature of the different bands of IgG was demonstrated by their relative ratio of κ/λ light chain determinants. A monoclonal nature of bands of IgG was previously shown by electrophoretic separation of CSF from cases of MS (17). The major clone of IgG occurring in the CSF shown in Fig. 9 represented antibodies against the nucleocapsid components. One somewhat more basic clone of IgG contained antibodies against the HL. Two additional clones of antibodies were found to be active in neutralizing, HLI and HI tests. These two clones displayed distinctly different electrophoretic mobilities. It has not as yet been demonstrated whether they represent antibodies, which react with the same or with different envelope components.

A possible preference for a certain virus component to induce the production of antibodies with a particular electrophoretic mobility was suggested from results of studies of samples from three additional cases of SSPE. One of these showed a distribution of IgG clones and antibody activities, which was strikingly similar to that of the sample illustrated in Fig. 9. Samples from the other two patients gave a less pronounced separation of clones by electrophoresis. However, different populations of specific antibodies displayed an electrophoretic mobility matching that of the corresponding antibodies in other samples. It is possible that the observed preference for clones carrying different antibody activities to display specific electrophoretic mobilities reflects the proposed (and experimentally demonstrated) inverse correlation between the net electrical charge of an antigen and the specific antibody against it (18).

THE SIGNIFICANCE OF ANTIBODIES AGAINST THE HEMOLYSIN OF MEASLES VIRUS IN PROTECTION AGAINST DISEASE

The occurrence of two biologically distinct envelope components, the hemagglutinin and the neuraminidase, at the surface of virions of orthomyxoviruses and most paramyxoviruses is well established. Paramyxoviruses in addition carry an HL. Certain properties of this HL have been described, but its true nature remains to be elucidated; measles virus, which carries an HL of similar characteristics, differs from most other paramyxoviruses in that it does not display any demonstrable neuraminidase activity (19). The neuraminidase and the HL of myxoviruses appear to serve different biological functions. It has been suggested that whereas neuraminidase may be of importance for the release of virus particles from cells (20,21), the HL of measles virions may play a role in the penetration of virus into cells (22). In spite of the distinct

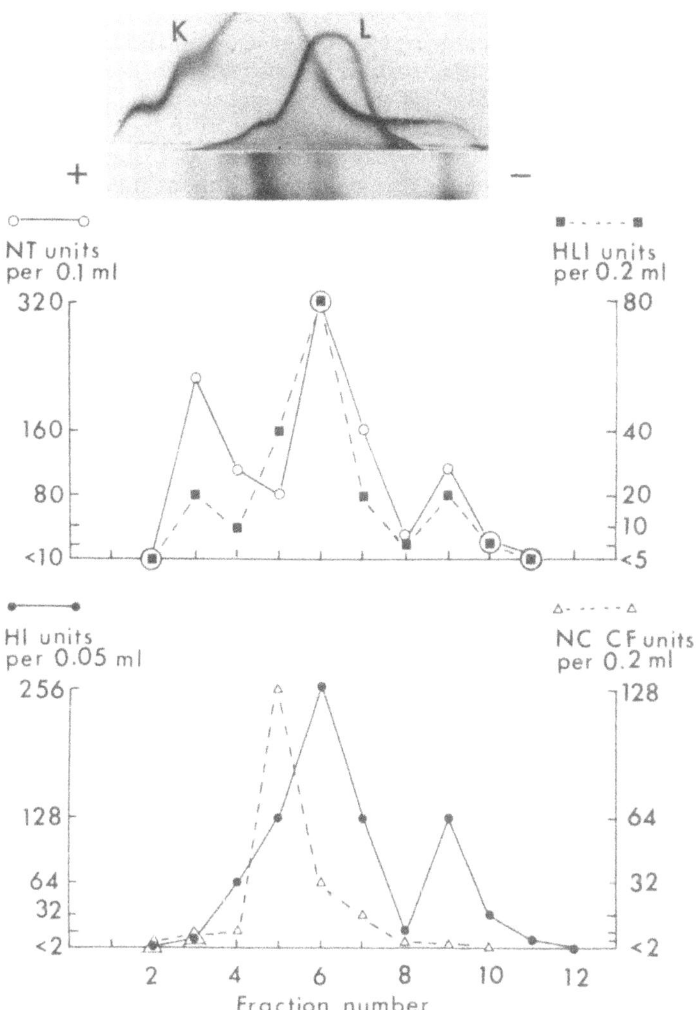

Fig. 9 Separation by preparative agarose gel electrophoresis of clones of IgG in concentrated CSF from a patient (R.S.) with SSPE. Antibodies were determined by the following tests: neutralization (o——o), HLI (■---■), HI (●——●) and nucleocapsid CF (Δ---Δ). The uppermost part of the figure shows the superimposed patterns of two crossed electrophoresis separations into gels containing antisera against human κ and λ light chains determinants, respectively. Note the monoclonal character of the various populations of IgG molecules with different electrophoretic mobilities.

biological characteristics of these two kinds of envelope components, it might be of interest to compare the effect on virion activities of antibodies against them. Antibodies against neuraminidase carry a certain capacity to inhibit hemagglutination by influenza virions (23). Similarly, antibodies against the HL of measles virus were found to be capable of blocking the agglutinating activity of crude, but not of Tween 80-ether-treated antigen. Antineuraminidase antibodies carry no direct neutralizing activity, but can sensitize virions (24). In contrast, antibodies against the measles virus HL gave a direct neutralization (cf. Fig. 9). As regards effects *in vivo*, it is known that under controlled experimental conditions, antineuraminidase antibodies may give protection against influenza, presumably by limiting the dissemination of the virus infection (25). The relative significance of antineuraminidase antibodies for protection against the disease in man has not been fully evaluated. It is known that relatively few individuals developed antibodies to the neuraminidase of A_2/1957 influenza virus on their first contact with this strain, but that after re-exposure to the virus these antibodies were demonstrable.

The importance of HLI antibodies for protection against measles in human beings is a matter for speculation. The frequency of development of HLI antibodies cannot be determined at present. The technical problem encountered is related to the fact that the presence of HI antibodies precludes the demonstration of HLI antibodies, unless the latter occur in a significantly higher titer. Therefore, a test has to be designed in which HI antibodies do not interfere with the identification of HLI antibodies, or HI antibodies have to be removed by absorption with purified HA before testing for HLI antibodies.

A discussion of a possible role of measles HLI antibodies for protection against the disease is of particular interest in relationship to any evaluation of the usefulness of inactivated measles vaccines. It has been found that the inactivated vaccines previously employed may induce the production of high titers of neutralizing and HI antibodies. However, these antibodies do not give the same protection as the corresponding amount of neutralizing and HI antibodies administered in the form of gamma globulin (26). This difference cannot be explained by reference to a lack of local production of IgA antibodies in the respiratory tract, since antibodies of this kind are absent in both situations. The most direct way of explaining the observed difference is to postulate that gamma globulin contains certain virus-specific antibodies, which are not produced by immunization with available inactivated vaccines. Antibodies against the HL might be of interest in this connection.

It has been demonstrated that after treatment with Tween 80 and ether no demonstrable hemolytic activity remains (1). This may be due either to destruction of the HL or to dissociation between the HL and HA components, since the activity of the former becomes expressed only when associated with HA. Experiments were carried out to determine the relative sensitivity of different biological activities to treatment with formalin, which is the main technique employed in the preparation of inactivated measles vaccine. It was found that the hemolysin activity was much more readily destroyed than the HA activity (Table 4).

TABLE IV

THE EFFECT OF FORMALIN ON THE HA AND HL ACTIVITIES OF RAPIDLY SEDIMENTING EXTRACELLULAR VIRUS PRODUCTS[(a)]

Type of Treatment	Time of Incubation at 37°C (Hours)	HA Activity (Units per 0.05 ml)	HL Activity (Units per 0.4 ml)
3.7% Formalin	0	150	24
" "	0.5	98	< 2
" "	2	48	< 2
Control	0	202	84
"	2	150	24

(a) Rapidly sedimenting extracellular virus products were prepared by centrifugation in discontinuous sucrose gradients (Fig. 3). Formalin in a final concentration of 3.7 percent or physiological saline (controls) was added and the samples incubated at 37°C for a predetermined time. Thereafter, rapidly sedimenting extracellular virus products were again isolated by centrifugation in discontinuous sucrose gradients. The accumulated values of HA and HL activities of fractions containing these products are given in the table.

As in the case of Tween 80-ether treatment, this can be explained as a destructive or dissociating effect of formalin, of which the destructive effect seems to be the more likely. Thus it seems possible that the two types of inactivated measles vaccines which have been studied, lack the capacity to induce production of HLI antibodies. An absence of antibodies of this kind might explain the poor capacity of these vaccines to confer protection against the disease. A comparative analysis of the occurrence of HLI antibodies in individuals who have had ordinary measles or who have been immunized with live or killed measles vaccines is highly warranted. However, as was already mentioned, it remains to develop a technique for separate identification of antibodies against the HL.

ACKNOWLEDGEMENTS

This work was supported by grants from the Swedish Medical Research Council (Project No. B71-16X-116-07), the National Research Council for Medical Sciences, Finland, the Finnish Medical Society "Duodecim" and the Norwegian Multiple Sclerosis Society.

B. Vandvik is a Fellow of the Norwegian Research Council for Science and the Humanities.

The skillful technical assistance of Miss Ylva Gollmar is gratefully acknowledged.

REFERENCES

1. NORRBY, E. *Arch. Gesamte Virusforsch.* *14:*306, 1964.
2. NORRBY, E. *Proc. Soc. Exp. Biol. Med.* *121:*948, 1966.
3. NUMAZAKI, Y. & KARZON, D.T. *J. Immunol.* *97:*458, 1966a.
4. NUMAZAKI, Y. & KARZON, D.T. *J. Immunol.* *97:*470, 1966b.
5. SCHLUEDERBERG, A. & ROIZMAN, B. *Virology* *16:*80, 1962.
6. WATERSON, A.P., ROTT, R. & RUCKLE-ENDERS, G. *Z. Naturforsch.* *18b:*378, 1963.
7. NORRBY, E. & HAMMARSKJÖLD, B. *Microbios.* (In press).
8. NORRBY, E. *Proc. Soc. Exp. Biol. Med.* *111:*814, 1962.
9. NORRBY, E. & GOLLMAR, Y. The appearance and persistence of antibodies against different virus components after regular measles infections. (1972) (To be published.)
10. SALMI, A.A., NORRBY, E. & PANELIUS, M. Identification of different measles virus-specific antibodies in the serum and cerebrospinal fluid from patients with subacute sclerosing panencephalitis and multiple sclerosis. (1972) (To be published.)

11. HENLE, G., HARRIS, S. & HENLE, W. *J. Exp. Med.* *88:*133, 1948.
12. BARBANTI-BRODANO, G., DYANAGI, S., KATZ, M. & KOPROWSKI, H. *Proc. Soc. Exp. Biol. Med.* *134:*230, 1970.
13. CONNOLLY, I.H. *Neurology* *18:*87, 1968.
14. NORRBY, E. van der VEEN, J. & ESPMARK, Å. *Proc. Soc. Exp. Biol. Med.* *134:*889, 1970.
15. PANELIUS, M., SALMI, A.A., HALONEN, P. & PENTTINEN, K. *Acta Neurol. Scand.* *47:*315, 1971.
16. VANDVIK, B. & NORRBY, E. Antibody activities of monoclonal IgG produced in the central nervous system of patients with subacute sclerosing panencephalitis. (1972) (To be published.)
17. ZETTERVALL, O & LINK, H. *Clin. Exp. Immunol.* *7:*365, 1970.
18. SELA, M. & MOZES, E. *Proc. Nat. Acad. Sci.* *55:*445, 1966.
19. HOWE, C. & SCHLUEDERBERG, A. *Biochim. Biophys. Res. Comm.* *40:*606, 1970.
20. SETO, J.T. & ROTT, R. *Virology* *30:*731, 1966.
21. WEBSTER, R.G. & LAVER, W.G. *J. Immunol.* *99:*49, 1967.
22. NORRBY, E. *Virology* *44:*599, 1971.
23. KILBOURNE, E.D., LAVER, W.G., SCHULMAN, J.L. & WEBSTER, R.G. *J. Virol.* *2:*281, 1968.
24. MAJER, M. & LINK, F. *J. Gen. Virol.* *13:*355, 1971.
25. SCHULMAN, J.L., KHAKPOUR, M. & KILBOURNE, E.D. *J. Virol.* *2:*778, 1968.
26. NORRBY, E. *PAHO Sci. Publ.* *147:*301, 1967.

STRUCTURAL AND IMMUNOLOGIC CHARACTERISTICS OF SUBVIRAL COMPONENTS OF SINDBIS, EASTERN EQUINE AND WESTERN EQUINE ENCEPHALITIS VIRUSES

N. Goldblum, R. Ravid, Amalia Hanoch and Yael Porath

Department of Virology
Hebrew University-Hadassah Medical School
Jerusalem, Israel

During recent years great progress has been made in the elucidation of the structure, composition and molecular properties of the arbovirion. It has been demonstrated that certain members of group A arboviruses-Sindbis and Semliki Forest - can be adequately purified and their subviral components separated and isolated in pure form. These viruses are composed of two major subviral constituents: a ribonucleoprotein core and a lipoprotein envelope (1-3).

We have developed procedures for the purification of the Sindbis virion and for the separation and characterization of its major subviral constituents (4,5). The present study deals with the separation of subviral components of Sindbis, Eastern Equine Encephalitis (E.E.E.) and Western Equine Encephalitis (W.E.E.) viruses, and the characterization of certain immunological properties of these constituents. Detailed procedures were reported previously (4,5).

Acrylamide gel electrophoresis of Sindbis subvirions labeled with radioactive amino acids (Fig. 1) showed the presence of one protein species (protein No. 1). A second protein (No. 2) with a higher molecular weight was also found in small quantity. Electrophoresis of the mature Sindbis virions demonstrated two proteins: (a) protein No. 1, which was present in the subvirions, and (b) a second protein (No. 2), which was incorporated into the virions during the maturation process. Protein No. 2 thus constitutes the protein component of the Sindbis virion envelope. This was demonstrated by electrophoresis in acrylamide gel of Sindbis virus labeled with ^{3}H-leucine and ^{14}C-glucosamine (Fig. 2). The two

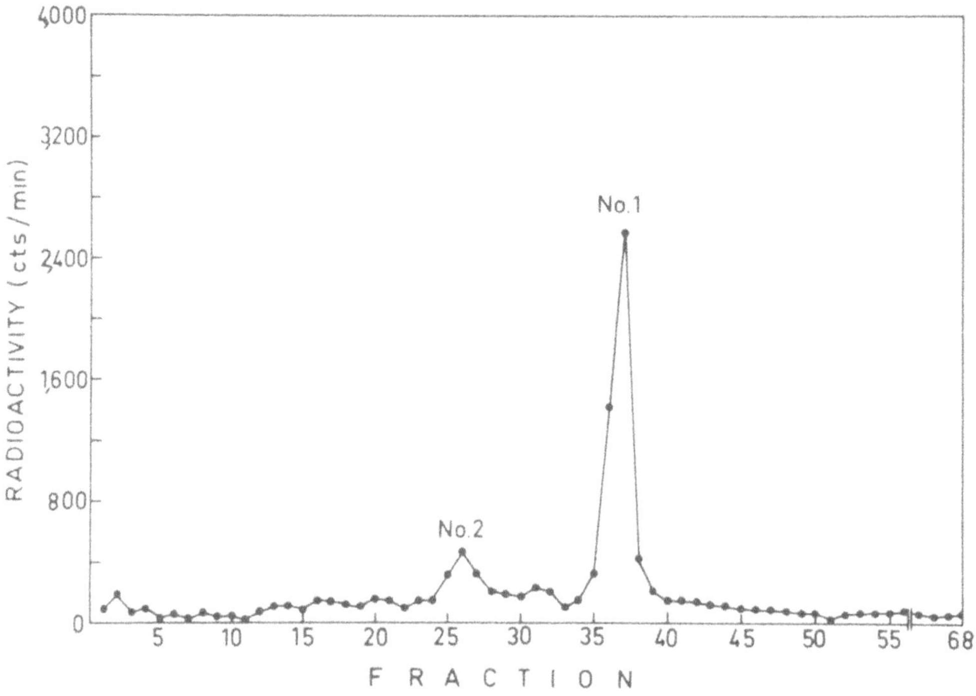

Fig. 1 Acrylamide gel electrophoresis of Sindbis subvirions labeled with aminoacids, showing protein No. 1; protein No. 2 of higher molecular weight is found in small quantity.

viral proteins are located by the ^{3}H-leucine label. In addition, protein No. 2 is also labeled with ^{14}C-glucosamine. This would indicate that the viral envelope is of a glycoprotein nature. These findings are in accord with those of Strauss *et al* (1).

The non-ionic detergent, Nonidet P-40, was used to separate the ribonucleoprotein core from the viral envelope. Following treatment of purified Sindbis virus overnight at 4°C with a 0.1 percent solution of Nonidet P-40, the suspension was banded in a sucrose gradient (15-30 percent w/w). The results are shown in Fig. 3.

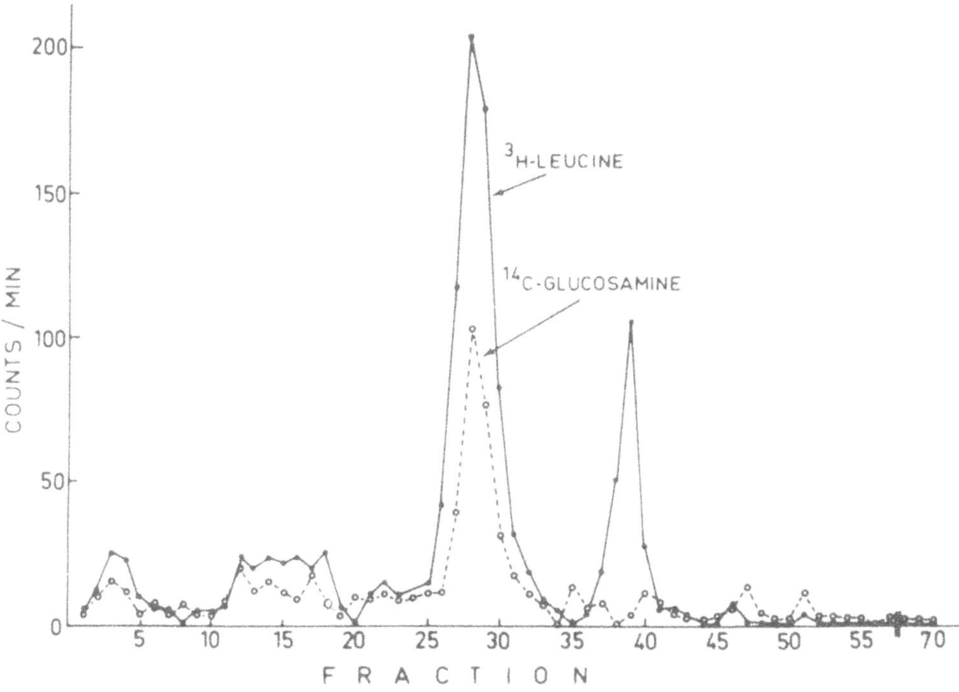

Fig. 2 Electrophoresis in acrylamide gel of Sindbis virus labeled with ^{3}H-leucine and ^{14}C-glucosamine.

Treatment with Nonidet P-40 resulted in the separation of Sindbis virions into a ribonucleoprotein core (peak labeled with ^{14}C-protein hydrolysate) and a viral envelope labeled with ^{3}H-choline (top of the gradient). This technique turned out to be very convenient for the separation of the two viral components, the ribonucleoprotein (RNP) core and lipoprotein (LP) envelope, and was subsequently used for the separation of the subviral components of E.E.E. and W.E.E. viruses and in all immunological tests and procedures. Occasionally, the RNP core was re-banded in sucrose with essentially similar results.

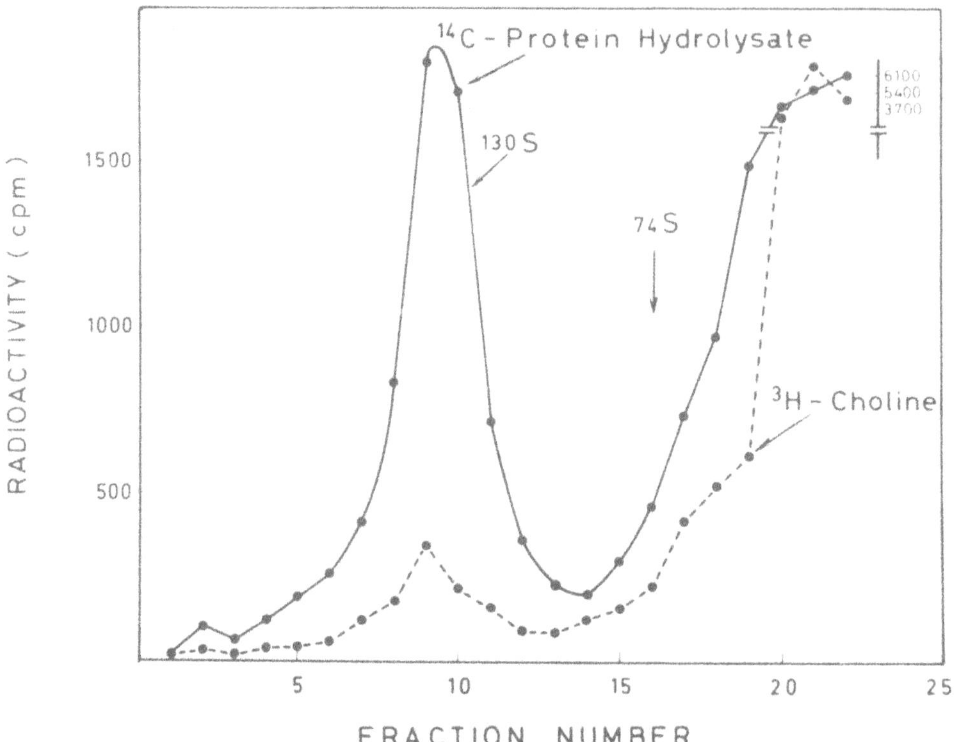

Fig. 3 Treatment with Nonidet P-40, resulting in the separation of Sindbis virions into a RNP core (labeled with protein hydrolysate), and a viral envelope LP (labeled with ^{3}H-choline).

Figures 4 to 7 present some data on the structure and composition of E.E.E. and W.E.E. viruses. Figure 4 demonstrates the separation of purified virions of E.E.E. virus into ribonucleoprotein core and viral envelope by use of the non-ionic detergent NP-40, following banding in a sucrose gradient. An almost identical profile was obtained for W.E.E. virions. Acrylamide gel electrophoresis of the separated RNP core and the viral envelope of W.E.E. are shown in Figs. 5 and 6 respectively, and that of virions labeled with both ^{3}H-leucine and ^{14}C-glucosamine in Fig. 7.

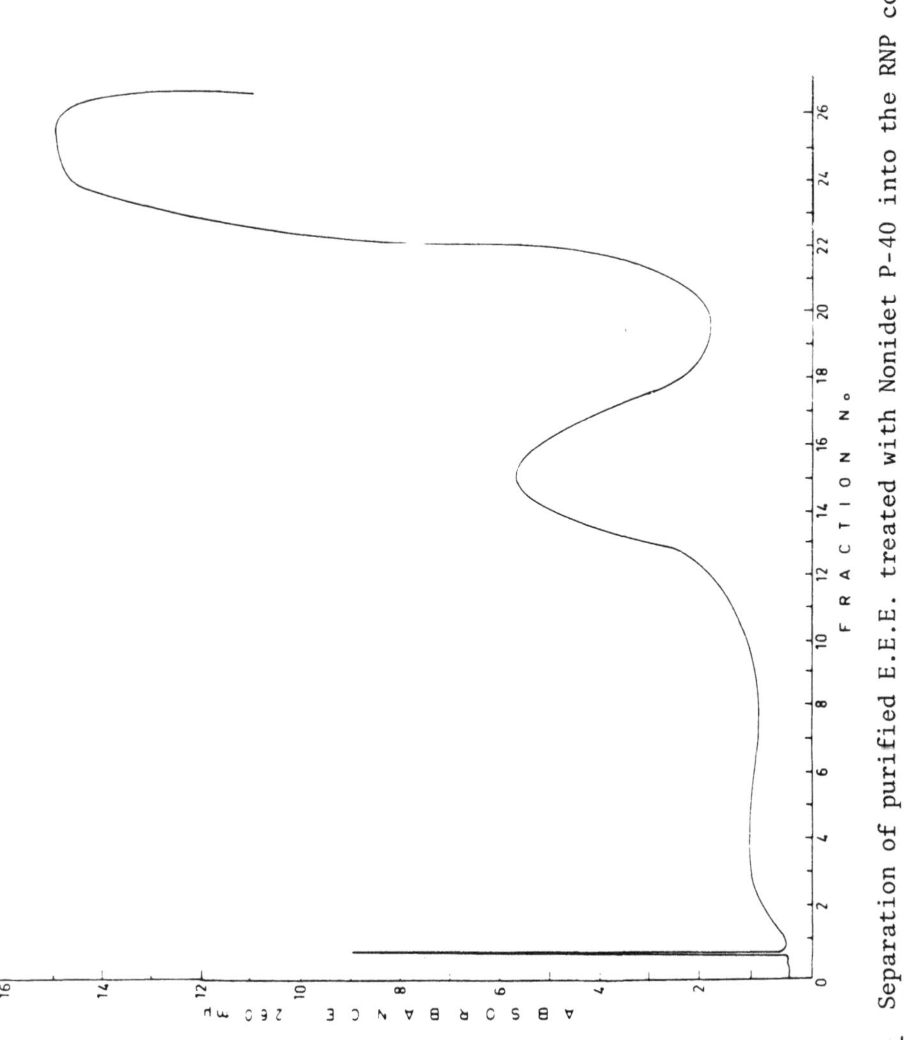

Fig. 4 Separation of purified E.E.E. treated with Nonidet P-40 into the RNP core (fraction 15) and LP envelope (top of gradient).

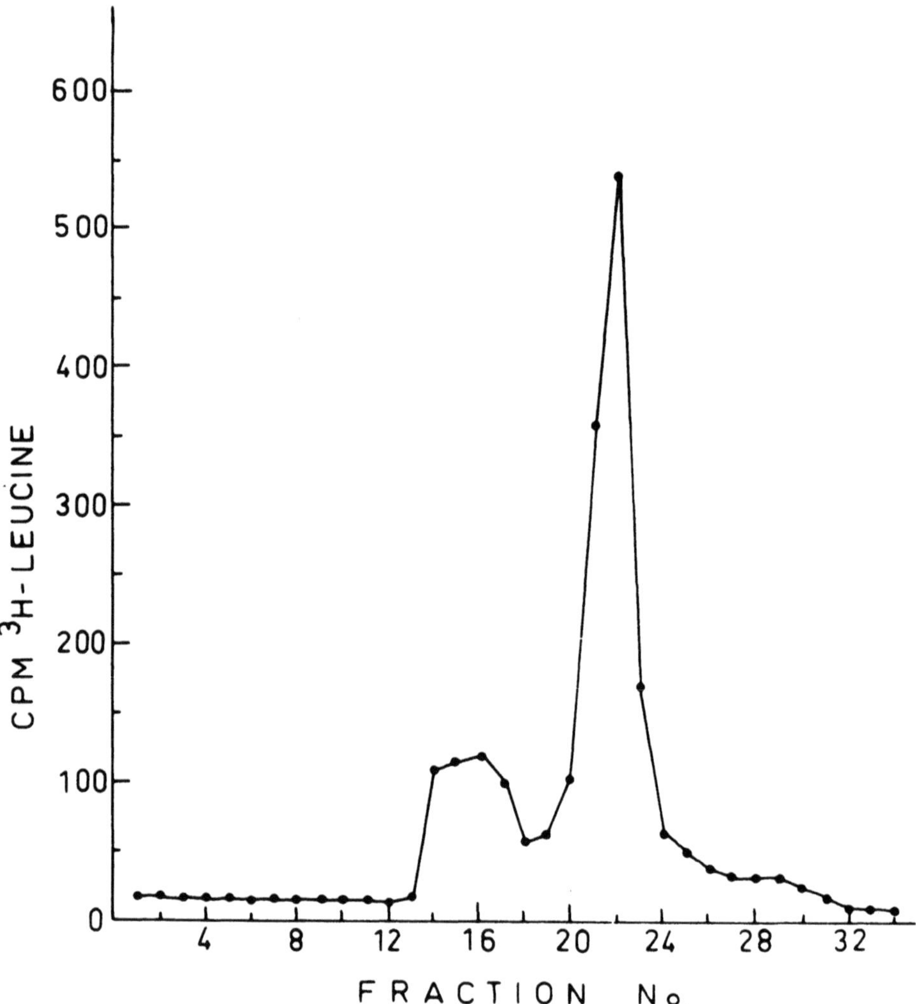

Fig. 5 Acrylamide gel electrophoresis of the separated RNP core of W.E.E.

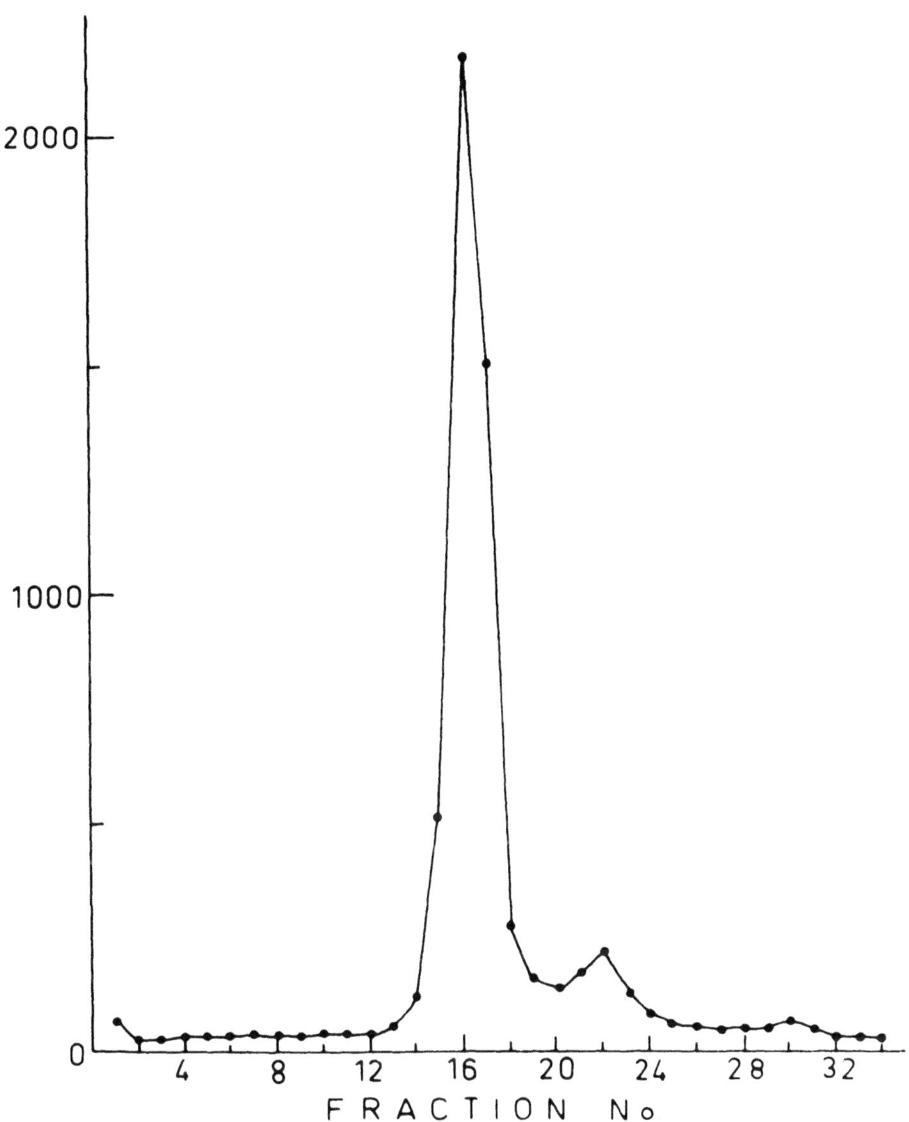

Fig. 6 Acrylamide gel electrophoresis of the separated envelope of W.E.E.

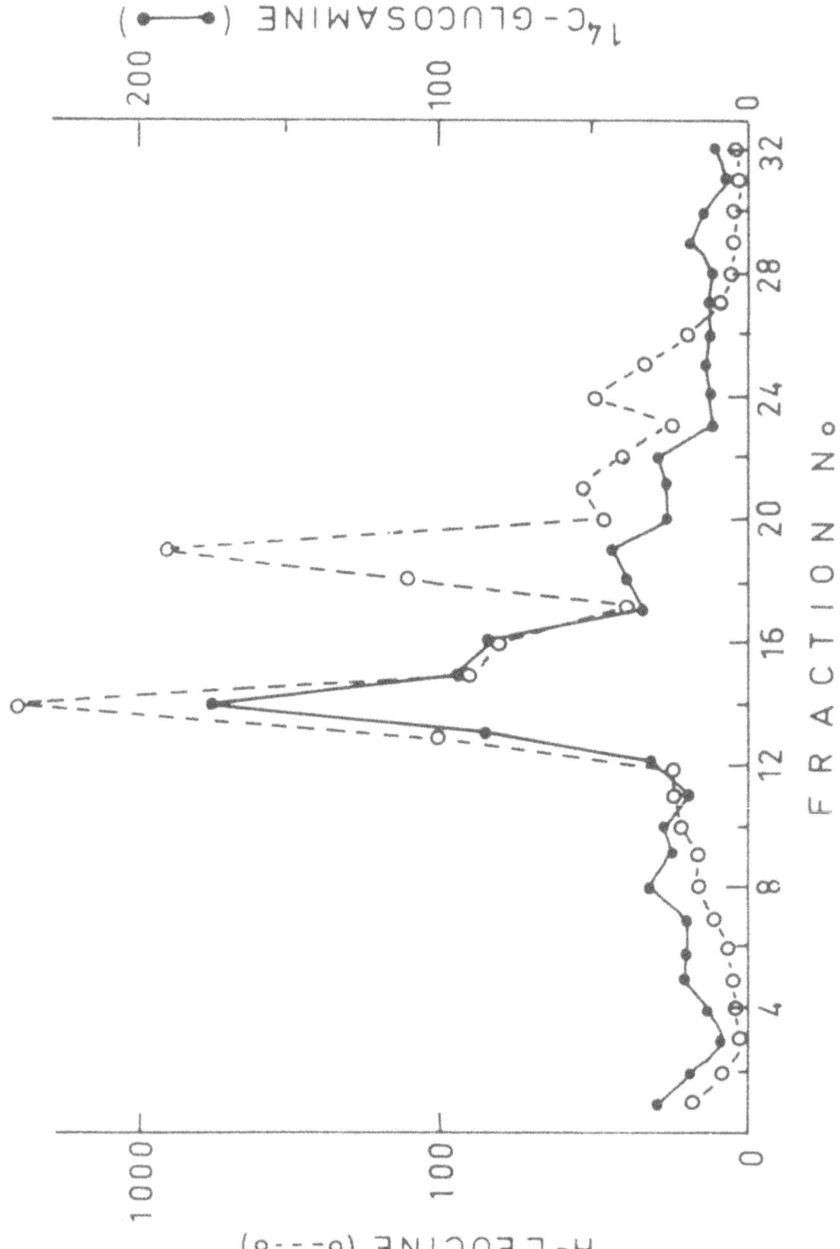

Fig. 7 Acrylamide gel electrophoresis of purified W.E.E. labeled with ^{3}H-leucine and ^{14}C-glucosamine.

In order to gain a better insight into the identity of the structure of Sindbis, E.E.E. and W.E.E. viruses, a series of co-electrophoresis runs was carried out, using pairs of viruses labeled with ^{14}C- and ^{3}H-leucine respectively. It is seen (Figs. 8a-c) that the profiles are almost identical.

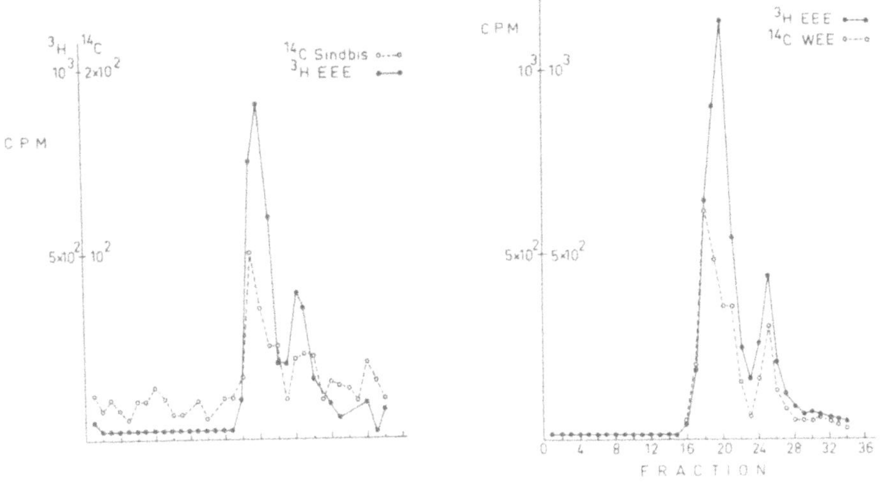

Fig. 8a Acrylamide gel electrophoresis of purified E.E.E. labeled with ^{3}H-leucine and Sindbis labeled with ^{14}C-leucine.

Fig. 8b Acrylamide gel electrophoresis of purified W.E.E. labeled with ^{14}C-leucine and E.E.E. labeled with ^{3}H-leucine.

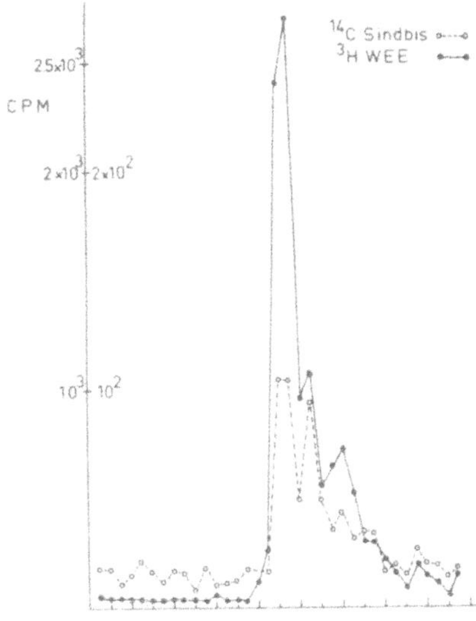

Fig. 8c Acrylamide gel electrophoresis of purified Sindbis virus labeled with ^{14}C-leucine and W.E.E. labeled with ^{3}H-leucine.

All these findings clearly indicate the great similarity in structure and composition of these virus types. If one adds to these data reported previously for Semliki Forest virus (2,3), and more recently for Semliki Forest (6) and Chikungunya virus (7), a highly uniform picture emerges of the structure and composition of group A arboviruses.

Immune sera to purified preparations of Sindbis virion, RNP core and LP envelope, respectively, were prepared in rabbits. The virion and subviral components were cross-tested with the immune sera in the gel diffusion, complement fixation, hemagglutination-inhibition and neutralization tests. Fig. 9 shows the results of the gel diffusion tests. The antigens (1-RNP core, 2-LP envelope and 3-virion) were diffused against anti-virion (a), anti-LP envelope (b) and anti-RNP core (c) sera. Three distinct antigenic components can be observed. Some crossing is apparent between virion and RNP and virion and LP, but none between RNP and LP. The complement fixation (CF) test also exhibited great specificity (Table 1). Immune serum against the virion gave high CF titers with virion, RNP and LP antigens. However, antisera prepared against the RNP and LP were highly specific, reacting almost solely with their homologous antigens.

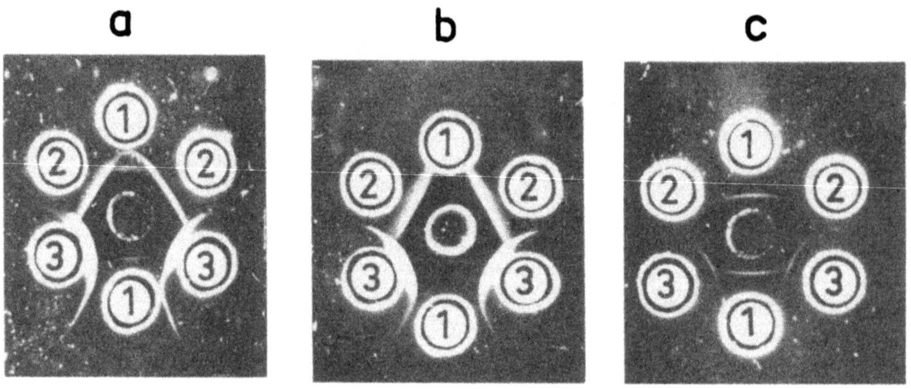

Fig. 9 Gel diffusion tests.

1 - RNP core
2 - LP envelope
3 - Virion
a - Antivirion serum
b - Anti LP serum
c - Anti RNP serum

TABLE I

COMPLEMENT FIXATION OF SINDBIS ANTIGENS WITH RABBIT IMMUNE SERA

Antigen	Rabbit Immune Sera Against:		
	Virion	Viral Envelope	Viral Core
Virion	4096	128	<32
Viral envelope	4096	1024	32
Viral core	4096	0	2048

The hemagglutinin (HA) was associated with the viral envelope. Fig. 10 shows a Sindbis virus preparation banded in sucrose, following overnight treatment with Nonidet P-40 (see also Fig. 3). The fractions from the gradient were tested for their HA titer. The results demonstrate that very little HA is present in the fractions containing the RNP core; the HA appears at the top of the gradient, associated with the viral LP envelope (Table 2). High hemagglutination-inhibition (HI) titers were found in the antisera prepared against the virion and the LP envelopes. Almost no HI was found in antisera prepared against the RNP core (Table 3). The neutralizing (NT) capacity of the immune sera, as measured by the extinction of plaque inhibition, was found to be confined mainly to the virion and LP envelope, almost to the same degree, with very little NT activity present in the antiserum prepared against the RNP core (Table 4).

The results of these serologic tests are very clear cut. They demonstrate the presence of at least three distinct antigens in the virion and respective antibodies in the immune sera. The gel diffusion and CF reactions show distinctly the specificity of these antigen-antibody reactions. The HA is undoubtedly a function of the viral envelope; the HI and NT antibodies are induced by the viral envelope. One wonders what is the immunological "function" of the RNP core, since high titer CF antibody against it is present in immune sera prepared against the virion. Further studies are needed to elucidate its immunologic role.

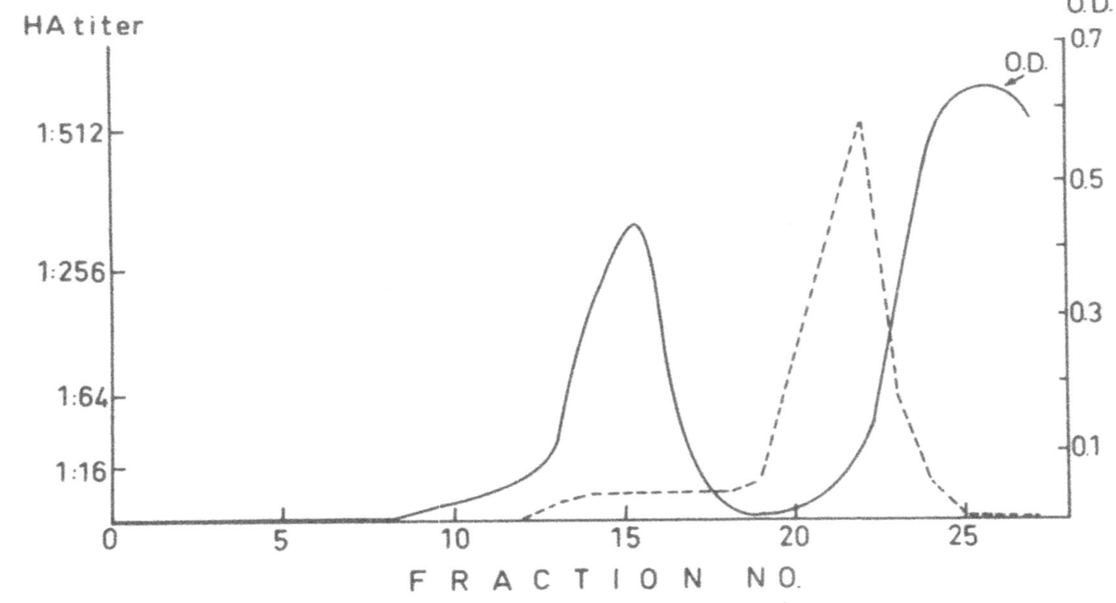

Fig. 10 Sucrose gradient of Sindbis virus treated with Nonidet P-40, demonstrating association of hemagglutinin with viral envelope.

—— Optical density

------ Hemagglutinin titer

TABLE II

HEMAGGLUTINATION (HA) TITER OF SINDBIS VIRION AND VIRAL COMPONENTS

Antigen	HA Titer
Virion	5120
Viral envelope	2560
Viral core	<2-8

TABLE III

HEMAGGLUTINATION-INHIBITION (HI) BY RABBIT IMMUNE SERA OF SINDBIS VIRION AND VIRAL COMPONENTS

HA Antigen	Rabbit Immune Sera Against:		
	Virion	Viral Envelope	Viral Core
Virion	2560-5120	640	<10-40
Viral envelope	2560-5120	320-1280	40-60

TABLE IV

PLAQUE INHIBITION OF SINDBIS VIRUS BY RABBIT IMMUNE SERA PREPARED AGAINST THE VIRION AND VIRAL COMPONENTS

Serum Dilution	Percent P.F.U. Inhibited by Rabbit Immune Sera Prepared Against:		
	Virion	Viral Envelope	Viral Core
1:10	100	100	83
1:100	100	92	0
1:400	93	78	0

Rabbit immune sera were also prepared to purified preparations of E.E.E. and W.E.E. virions, envelopes and cores. All these preparations are presently being tested in homologous and heterologous immune cross-reactions. Results of a representative cross HI is shown in Table 5. The homologous HI reactions of E.E.E. exhibit a pattern similar to that of Sindbis (see Table 3); more extensive tests are needed to enable a more precise interpretation of the heterologous immune reactions to be made.

We have lately carried out "further splitting" of the subviral components - the core and especially the envelope - using proteolytic enzymes, such as pronase and trypsin, as well as glycosidases such as neuraminidase and β-galactosidase. The immunogenicity of these preparations and their direct and indirect behavior in the various serologic reactions is at present under study.

TABLE V

CROSS HEMAGGLUTINATION-INHIBITION BETWEEN E.E.E. VIRION AND IMMUNE SERA TO VIRION AND VIRAL COMPONENTS OF E.E.E., SINDBIS AND W.E.E.

HA Antigen	Immune Serum Against:	HI Titer
E.E.E. virion	E.E.E. virion	1280
	E.E.E. envelope	320-640
	E.E.E. core	20
	Sindbis virion	160-320
	Sindbis envelope	40
	Sindbis core	< 20
	W.E.E. virion	< 20
Sindbis virion	Sindbis virion	2560
	E.E.E. virion	160

REFERENCES

1. STRAUSS, J.H., BURGE, B.W., PFEFFERKORN, E.R. & DARNELL, J.E. *Proc. Nat. Acad. Sci.* *60:*533, 1968.
2. FRIEDMAN, R.M. *J. Virol.* *2:*1076, 1968.
3. HAY, A.J., SHEKEL, J.J. & BURKE, D.C. *J. Gen. Virol.* *3:*175, 1968.
4. BEN-ISHAI, Z., GOLDBLUM, N. & BECKER, Y. *J. Gen. Virol.* *2:* 365, 1968.
5. GOLDBLUM, N., RAVID, ZOHAR, BEN-ISHAI, Z. & BECKER, Y. PAHO/WHO International Conference, Washington, D.C., 14-18 December, 1970.
6. APPLEYARD, G., ORAN, J.D. & STANLEY, J.L. *J. Gen. Virol.* *9:* 179, 1970.
7. IGARASHI, A., FUKUOKA, T., NITHIUTHAI, P., HSU, L. & FUKAI, K. *Biken Journal* *13:*93, 1970.

SECRETORY AND SYSTEMIC CELL-MEDIATED AND HUMORAL IMMUNE RESPONSE IN HUMANS AND GUINEA PIGS TO THE INACTIVATED INFLUENZA VIRUS VACCINE

R.H. Waldman, N. Gadol, P.F. Jurgensen, G.N. Olsen and J.E. Johnson, III

University of Florida College of Medicine
Gainesville, Florida, U.S.A.

In the past few years, there has been a great deal of interest in what has been called the secretory immunologic system (1-6). A stimulus has been the basic immunologic finding that the predominant immunoglobulin in external secretions is secretory IgA, i.e., dimerized IgA containing secretory component (6-8). However, in 1927, Besredka (9) had already described his work and the work of others on the production of immunity against pathogens of the gastrointestinal tract by direct stimulation through the feeding of antigens. Sporadic investigations of the secretory immunologic system ensued, but it was not until the mid 1960's that immunologists became greatly interested.

Several components do or may play a role in immunity on mucosal surfaces. One is secretory IgA. Others are IgG, IgM and IgD present in external secretions. Evidence indicates, however, that the latter immunoglobulins reach the lumina of secretory organs primarily by simple diffusion, that is, very little is produced locally (10). This is not true of IgE; large numbers of IgE-producing cells line the respiratory and gastrointestinal tracts (11), and IgE is found in external secretions in amounts larger than one would expect as a result of simple diffusion (12). It would seem reasonable to assume that IgE in respiratory secretions may play a role in the prevention, and/or pathogenesis of respiratory disease, including viral respiratory diseases. The inter-relationship between IgA and IgE in secretions is an intriguing one, and there is one study (13) which suggests that IgE is more important in protection of the respiratory tract against infections than is IgA, but this has not been confirmed.

Secretory antibody is produced locally in the secretory mucosa. Most of the antibodies to *Herpesvirus hominis* in lacrimal secretions (14), to respiratory syncytial virus (15) rhinovirus (16), parainfluenza virus (17,18), poliovirus (19), influenza virus (20,21) and diphtheria toxoid (22) in respiratory secretions, to cholera vibrio cell-wall antigens (23) in the gastrointestinal secretions, and to *Candida albicans* antigens in the female genital tract (24), to name a few, have been shown to be IgA immunoglobulins. In many of these studies, subcutaneous immunization has been shown to stimulate serum antibody to virtually the same level as actual infection; however, this route of immunization stimulated little secretory antibody.

In studies with influenza virus, neither subcutaneous immunization nor local application of infective or inactivated virus was very efficient in stimulating neutralizing antibody activity in saliva, an external secretion similar to nasal secretions or sputum, with regard to content of secretory IgA (25,26). This lends support to the hypothesis that secretory IgA antibody is locally produced and stimulated, since the salivary glands are not stimulated directly by antigen during influenza infection or following aerosol or subcutaneous immunization.

One antibody-producing site of the secretory IgA system probably is not induced to produce specific antibody following application of antigen to another site, although this is somewhat controversial. As mentioned, antibody production in nasal secretions and sputum was not accompanied by a corresponding response in saliva. Ogra and Karzon (27) have reported that when poliovirus antigen was introduced into one limb of the large intestine in patients with double colonic stomas, specific antibody was produced in that limb, but not elsewhere. Antibody response in nasal secretion is better if influenza virus vaccine is administered into the upper rather than the lower respiratory tract. The converse is true for antibody in sputum (21). This suggests that secretory IgA antibody is produced locally when antigen is applied to that site.

Several studies have shown that parenterally administered antigens stimulate the production of secretory antibody, but not as efficiently as does local application of antigen. Killed influenza virus (20,21,26),parainfluenza virus (18), poliovirus (19), rhinovirus (16), diphtheria toxoid (22), and tetanus toxoid (28) given subcutaneously stimulate high levels of serum antibody but much lower levels of antibody in respiratory secretion than does local application of antigen.

The presence of IgA antibody in respiratory secretion and protection against infection are not necessarily synonymous. To test the ability of antibody to protect, field trials of aerosol immunization in influenza epidemics have been carried out. In three trials (29-31), the aerosol route rendered protection rates of 70 to 80 percent. The primary differences noted among these three field trials involved the protection rates afforded by subcutaneous immunization.

The presence of secretory IgA antibody is correlated with protection against illness, as is indicated by studies with rhinovirus (32) and parainfluenza virus (33) which showed that the antibody in nasal secretion is more closely related to protection than that in serum antibody.

However, this relationship between secretory IgA antibody and protection may not be a direct one in all cases: it may be simply an indirect indication of some other host defence mechanism, much as probably serum antibody is, in the cases where protection against various virus respiratory infections has been shown to correlate roughly with serum antibody titers (34,35). One host defence mechanism that may play a role on secretory surfaces, and one that is undergoing intense investigation at the present time, is interferon.

Another host defence mechanism that is known to play an important role in protection against viral infections is cell-mediated immunity (CMI), i.e., that form of immunity which depends on the specific activity of thymus-derived lymphocytes and which may act through an effector cell, the macrophage. The relationship of CMI to protection against viral infections is largely based on the observation that humans with hypogamma-globulinemia have no greatly increased susceptibility to viral infections, whereas patients with a defect in CMI are much more susceptible.

With regard to secretory surfaces, recent data suggest that secretory IgA is not the only protective mechanism. The most impressive evidence comes from a study with volunteers which showed that protection can be afforded with an attenuated respiratory syncytial virus vaccine without the stimulation of either serum or secretory antibody (36). Some other mechanism, possibly CMI, must account for this protection.

Despite the fact that specifically sensitized lymphocytes which are active in cell-mediated immunity constitute a distinct mode of immune response, apparently independent of humoral antibodies, cell-mediated immunity on mucosal surfaces has not been studied to any significant degree. Studies were undertaken to investigate the cell-mediated and humoral immune response in guinea pigs to local and systemic immunization against influenza virus.

There were two variables in the immunization program: route and dosage. One group of animals received 0.1 ml of a 1:10 dilution of influenza virus vaccine by nose drops while the animals were lightly anesthetized (low-dose nasal group). A second group received 0.1 ml of the undiluted vaccine by nose drops (high-dose nasal group). The third and fourth groups received either the low dose or the high dose of vaccine mixed with 0.1 ml of complete Freund's adjuvant, administered parentally in the rear footpads (low dose parenteral and high dose parenteral groups). At various times after immunization, groups of animals were given a lethal dose of sodium pentobarbital intraperitoneally. When the animals were anesthetized but still living, the thoracic cavity was opened and they were exsanguinated by cardiac puncture. The blood was saved and the serum separated later for use in antibody determinations. The trachea was then clamped as cephalad as possible and cut above the clamp. The respiratory tract was removed from the body and washed (exteriorly) with saline; the clamp was removed, and the bronchial washings were obtained by lavaging, using a Pasteur pipette, with sterile Eagle's medium. This was accomplished by alternately instilling and aspirating in each main stem bronchus about 1 ml of Eagle's medium until a total of 5 ml of media had been instilled. The yield was usually 3.0 - 3.5 ml of cells and fluid. At the same time that the bronchial washings were being done, the spleen was removed from each animal.

Cell-mediated immunity was determined using the inhibition of macrophage migration test, according to the method of David (37). The application of this technique to cells obtained by bronchial washing has been previously reported (38). At a dose of influenza virus vaccine adjusted by weight equivalent to that used in human immunization, parenteral immunization led to the development of circulating antibody and to cell-mediated immunity, as determined by the inhibition of macrophage migration, in splenic lymphocytes. After immunization with nose drops, local cellular and humoral immunity developed but there was little systemic immunologic response. At a larger dose of antigen, equivalent to ten times the usual dose given to immunized humans, cell-mediated immunity developed in both the bronchial washing lymphocytes and the splenic lymphocytes in the parenterally immunized animals. Humoral immunity, however, maintained the same pattern as in the animals which received the lower dose of vaccine; i.e., locally immunized animals developed mainly local antibody and parenterally immunized animals developed mainly systemic antibody. The inhibition of macrophage migration activity had disappeared or was greatly reduced in both the splenic and bronchial wash lymphocytes by 28 days; however, the influenza-neutralizing antibody persisted through this time. Thus, cellular immunity in the bronchial washing cells was best stimulated by nose-drops immunization, whereas cellular immunity in the splenic cells was stimulated better by parenteral immunization (Table 1). In

TABLE I

INHIBITION OF MACROPHAGE MIGRATION*

	Route of Immunization			
	Nose Drops		Parental Administration into Footpads	
	Source of Lymphocytes			
	Bronchial Washings	Splenic	Bronchial Washings	Splenic
High-dose Group	58.3 ± 4.6	40.8 ± 8.2	64.0 ± 4.3	59.4 ± 4.2
Low-dose Group	37.4 ± 3.3	19.7 ± 3.8	19.6 ± 1.9	49.2 ± 2.3

*Mean of all determinations at 7, 14, 21 and 28 days after immunization (± standard error of the mean).

Values expressed as mean percent inhibition.

both the high-dose and the low-dose receiving animals, the development of antibody reflected the route of immunization. Antibody titers in serum and bronchial washings were significantly higher in the high-dose groups, regardless of route of administration.

The results suggest that the inhibition of macrophage migration by bronchial washing cells is not related to humoral antibody in that influenza virus neutralization activity in bronchial-washing fluid existed unabated at 28 days, while the inhibition of macrophage migration had virtually disappeared by 28 days. Thus, disappearance of the humoral and cellular immune responses, whether local or systemic, follow differing time courses.

Another study was undertaken to evaluate the secondary, as compared to the primary response, to evaluate the possible movement of sensitized lymphocytes from the spleen to the lung, and vice versa, and to compare the cellular and humoral immune responses. Guinea pigs were immunized with influenza virus vaccine either by nose drops or parenterally: booster immunizations were carried out either by the same or opposite route, and groups of 4-6 animals were sacrificed at various times following immunization. As in previous studies, local application of antigen led to mainly a local appearance of CMI, whereas parenteral immunization led to mainly systemic CMI. Both pulmonary and splenic lymphocytes showed an IMM response that appeared sooner (2-3 days) and persisted longer, following the booster, than did the response to the primary immunization. Similarly, antibody in the bronchial secretions appeared earlier in the "boosted" animals. In the "cross-boosted" animals, CMI appeared in a fashion similar to the primary response. The results indicate that pulmonary, as well as splenic, T- and B-lymphocytes exhibit memory, and that there is no significant movement of sensitized lymphocytes between the spleen and lung (Table 2).

The cellular and humoral immune responses to immunization with influenza virus vaccine either subcutaneously or by aerosol were studied in humans. Bronchoalveolar (BA) lavage, nasal washing and venopuncture were carried out on 21 volunteers before and after immunization. Cell-mediated immunity was assessed by studying the inhibition of macrophage migration (IMM) using the BA lymphocytes, and determining the B-N-acetylglucosaminidase (BNAG) level of the alveolar macrophages as a measure of lysosomal acid hydrolase activity. Immunoglobulin and antibody levels were measured of the supernatants of the various body fluids.

The results indicate that the IgG:IgA ratios are different in the various body fluids studied: values of about 5:1 were found in serum, 1:2 in nasal secretions, and 3:1 in BA washings. Influenza neutralizing antibody titers in BA fluid and in nasal washings were highest following aerosol immunization, with the mean titer rising five-fold in the BA fluid of volunteers immunized by aerosol, and three-fold in those immunized subcutaneously. The serum antibody titers, however, rose four-fold and 25-fold respectively. Following aerosol immunization, BA lymphocytes gave 30 percent inhibition in the IMM test, while circulating lymphocytes gave five percent inhibition. Following subcutaneous immunization, a reverse pattern was seen, with BA lymphocytes giving 16 percent inhibition, while circulating lymphocytes gave 28 percent inhibition (Table 3). The level of BNAG in alveolar macrophages rose significantly following aerosol, but not following subcutaneous immunization.

These data confirm and extend the results of several studies in recent years which indicate that the lower respiratory tract is a relatively independent immunologic organ.

TABLE II

MEAN MACROPHAGE MIGRATION INHIBITION IN GUINEA PIGS IMMUNIZED WITH INACTIVATED INFLUENZA VIRUS*

Immunization Route		Source of	Time (Days)					
First	Second	Lymphocytes	2-3	4-5	6-10	14-21	28-35	<35
Nasal	-	Spleen	0	11	35	8	7	5
		Lungs	0	19	42	53	14	0
Foot-pad	-	Spleen	3	16	52	49	24	0
		Lungs	0	1	18	24	6	0
Nasal	Nasal	Spleen	12	5	21	7	13	5
		Lungs	23	20	26	65	25	18
Foot-pad	Foot-pad	Spleen	24	29	26	52	14	27
		Lungs	10	12	15	32	5	11
Nasal	Foot-pad	Spleen	0	8	23	32	20	0
		Lungs	0	9	7	26	18	5
Foot-pad	Nasal	Spleen	0	3	17	24	6	1
		Lungs	0	21	26	39	25	11

*Mean percent inhibition

TABLE III

IMMUNE RESPONSES TO INFLUENZA IMMUNIZATION IN VOLUNTEERS

Route of Immunization	Mean Rise in Influenza Antibody			Mean IMM Percent Inhibition			
	Serum	Nasal	BA	Circulating		BA	
				Pre	Post	Pre	Post
Subcutaneous	25-fold	1	3	7	28	12	16
Aerosol	4	3	5	0	5	7	30

ACKNOWLEDGEMENT

This work was supported by NIH Grant AI10295-01 and The Irwin Strasburger Foundation.

REFERENCES

1. TOMASI, T.B., JR., BIENENSTOCK, J. *Adv. Immunol.* *9:*1, 1968.
2. SMALL, P.A., JR., WALDMAN, R.H. The Secretory Immunologic System. In Sterzl, J., Riha, I. (Editors): Proceedings of the International Symposium on the Developmental Aspects of Antibody Formation and Structure, p. 445. Prague, Academic Publishing House, 1970.
3. WALDMAN, R.H. *Am. J. Med. Sci.* *260:*255, 1970.
4. BIENENSTOCK, J. *Can. Med. Assoc. J.* *103:*39, 1970.
5. TOMASI, T.B., DE COTEAU, E. *Adv. Intern. Med.* *16:*401, 1970.
6. DAYTON, D.H., JR., SMALL, P.A., JR., CHANOCK, R.M. ET AL. (Editors): The Secretory Immunologic System. U.S. Department of Health, Education and Welfare, National Institutes of Health, National Institute of Child Health and Development, Washington, D.C., U.S. Government Printing Office, 1971.
7. HANSON, L.A. *Int. Arch. Allergy Appl. Immunol.* *18:*241, 1961.
8. TOMASI, T.B., JR., TAM, E.M., SOLOMON, A., ET AL. *J. Exp. Med.* *121:*101, 1965.
9. BESREDKA, A. Local Immunization. Baltimore, The Williams & Wilkins Company, 1927.
10. BUTLER, W.T., ROSSEN, R.D., WALDMANN, T.A. *J. Clin. Invest.* *46:*1883, 1967.
11. TADA, T., ISHIZAKA, K. *J. Immunol.* *104:*377, 1970.
12. ISHIZAKA, K., NEWCOMB, R.W. *J. Allergy* *46:*197, 1970.
13. HONG, R., AMMANN, A.J., CAIN, W.A., GOOD, R.A. *Ibid. 6*, p. 433.
14. CENTIFANTO, Y.M., KAUFMAN, H.E. *Ibid. 6*, p. 331.
15. PARROTT, R.H., KIM, H.W., BELLANTI, J.A., ET AL. *Ibid. 6*, p. 167.
16. KNOPF, H.L., PERKINS, J.C., BERTRAN, D.M. ET AL. *J. Immunol.* *104:*566, 1970.
17. SMITH, C.B., BELLANTI, J.A., CHANOCK, R.M. *J. Immunol.* *99:* 133, 1967.
18. WIGLEY, F.M., FRUCHTMAN, M.H., WALDMAN, R.H. *N. Engl. J. Med.* *283:*1250, 1970.
19. OGRA, P.L., KARZON, D.T. *J. Immunol.* *102:*15, 1969.
20. KASEL, J.A., HUME, E.B., FULK, R.V. ET AL. *J. Immunol.* *102:* 555, 1969.

21. WALDMAN, R.H., WOOD, S.H., TORRES, E.H. ET AL. *Am. J. Epidemiol. 91:*575, 1970.
22. NEWCOMB, R.W., ISHIZAKA, K., DE VALD, B.L. *J. Immunol. 103:* 215, 1969.
23. WALDMAN, R.H., BENCIC, Z., SAKAZAKI, R. ET AL. (To be published.)
24. WALDMAN, R.H., CRUZ, J.M., ROWE, D.S. *Clin. Exp. Immunol.* (in press).
25. MANN, J.J., WALDMAN, R.H., TOGO, Y. ET AL. *J. Immunol. 100:* 726, 1968.
26. WALDMAN, R.H., KASEL, J.A., FULK, R.V. ET AL. *Nature 218:* 594, 1968.
27. OGRA, P.L., KARZON, D.T. *J. Immunol. 102:*1423, 1969.
28. WIGLEY, F.M., WOOD, S.H., WALDMAN, R.H. *J. Immunol. 103:* 1096, 1969.
29. WALDMAN, R.H., MANN, J.J., SMALL, P.A., JR. *JAMA 207:*520, 1969.
30. WALDMAN, R.H., BOND, J.O., LEVITT, L.P., ET AL. *Bull. WHO 41:*543, 1969.
31. WALDMAN, R.H., COGGINS, W.J. *J. Inf. Dis.* (in press).
32. PERKINS, J.C., TUCKER, D.N., KNOPF, H.L.S., ET AL. *Am. J. Epidemiol. 90:*319, 1969.
33. SMITH, C.B., PURCELL, R.H., BELLANTI, J.A., ET AL. *N. Engl. J. Med. 275:*1145, 1966.
34. FRANCIS, T., JR. *Bull. N.Y. Acad. Med. 17:*268, 1941.
35. FRANCIS, T., JR. *The Harvey Lectures 37:*69, 1941.
36. CHANOCK, R.M. Progress in Immunology, p. 1244. Ed. by B. Amos, Academic Press, 1971.
37. DAVID, J.R. *Proc. Nat. Acad. Sci. U.S.A. 56:*72, 1966.
38. HENNEY, C.S., & WALDMAN, R.H. *Science 169:*696, 1970.

CONCEPTS OF LOUSE-BORNE TYPHUS CONTROL IN DEVELOPING COUNTRIES: THE USE OF THE LIVING ATTENUATED E STRAIN TYPHUS VACCINE IN EPIDEMIC AND ENDEMIC SITUATIONS

Charles L. Wisseman, Jr.

Department of Microbiology
University of Maryland School of Medicine
Baltimore, Maryland, U.S.A.

INTRODUCTION

Louse-borne or epidemic typhus fever is without doubt one of the great epidemic diseases of mankind whose ebb and flow through the centuries has been important in the molding of human destiny (1). Much of our knowledge about typhus fever has come from experience in the unique setting of the temperate north of Europe (1-16) where its relative importance has declined as living conditions have improved over many years. Indeed, in recent times the epidemic potential of typhus in Europe has been realized primarily in the wake of the catastrophic disruptions caused by wars. Our attitude about relative importance, epidemiology, approaches to control and level of research support has been influenced strongly by the trends in modern, advanced Europe.

However, there is another face to typhus, hardly mentioned in our textbooks, largely ignored by investigators and treated as an unwanted step-child by many health authorities, which may be readily seen today in the less developed areas of the world where huge numbers of human beings still live continuously under conditions which most of us would regard as catastrophic and where typhus is a problem. Indeed, at present typhus is endemic to a greater or lesser degree on all continents except Australia and it is epidemic on at least one.

An attempt, albeit brief, will be made here (a) to construct a conceptual framework of the natural history of typhus infections and then, in the context of this framework, (b) to describe the actual state of typhus in some developing countries, (c) to consider the applicability and limitations of available control methods under the conditions which exist in such areas and (d) to illustrate briefly how one of these methods, namely, immunization with the living attenuated E strain typhus vaccine, is being applied on a pilot, investigational scale in two contrasting epidemiologic situations, one epidemic and one endemic.

THE NATURAL HISTORY OF TYPHUS INFECTIONS: A SIMPLIFIED CONCEPTUAL MODEL

The particular epidemiologic pattern assumed by typhus in any given situation depends largely upon the interactions among the major variables in the system which are recognized as (a) the agent, *Rickettsia prowazeki* (4,5), (b) the vector, the body louse *Pediculus humanus humanus* L. (3), and (c) Man, who serves as host to both agent and vector, as a reservoir of the rickettsia and as a mobile agent whose behavior markedly influences the other variables and determines the particular pattern of transmission (2, 6-8). Interaction is stressed because in large, complex populations, it is possible for vector, agent in its reservoir and susceptible people to co-exist without interacting, as in the U.S.A. today.

In this brief discussion, we will not consider possible variations in properties of agent or vector, only quantitative variations in prevalence; nor can we dwell upon environmental factors, except as they interfere with the application of control measures. We will also ignore the possibility of extra-human reservoirs (17) which, if they do exist, have not yet been demonstrated to play any role in the transmission of disease to man.

Recognizing these restrictions, and ignoring for simplicity many other extremely interesting variables, it is possible to portray the major interactions diagrammatically, as in Figure 1, and to identify empirically several major and some minor epidemiological stages in the natural history of typhus which have both practical and theoretical value. Although other special situations are possible, most naturally-occurring typhus can be fitted into this scheme; the major factors leading to change in stage can be identified and the consequences of the application of specific control measures can be predicted. From the stand-point of typhus control, which is the main topic of this report, the two most vulnerable points of attack at any stage are clearly recognizable as (a) the vector, through vector control measures, and (b) the susceptible human population, through active immunization. This diagram also stresses the crucial role of the reservoir, i.e., the human typhus convalescent who later develops recrudescent (Brill-Zinsser) disease and the long-range consequences of permitting any transmission of agent to occur. We have no proven means yet of

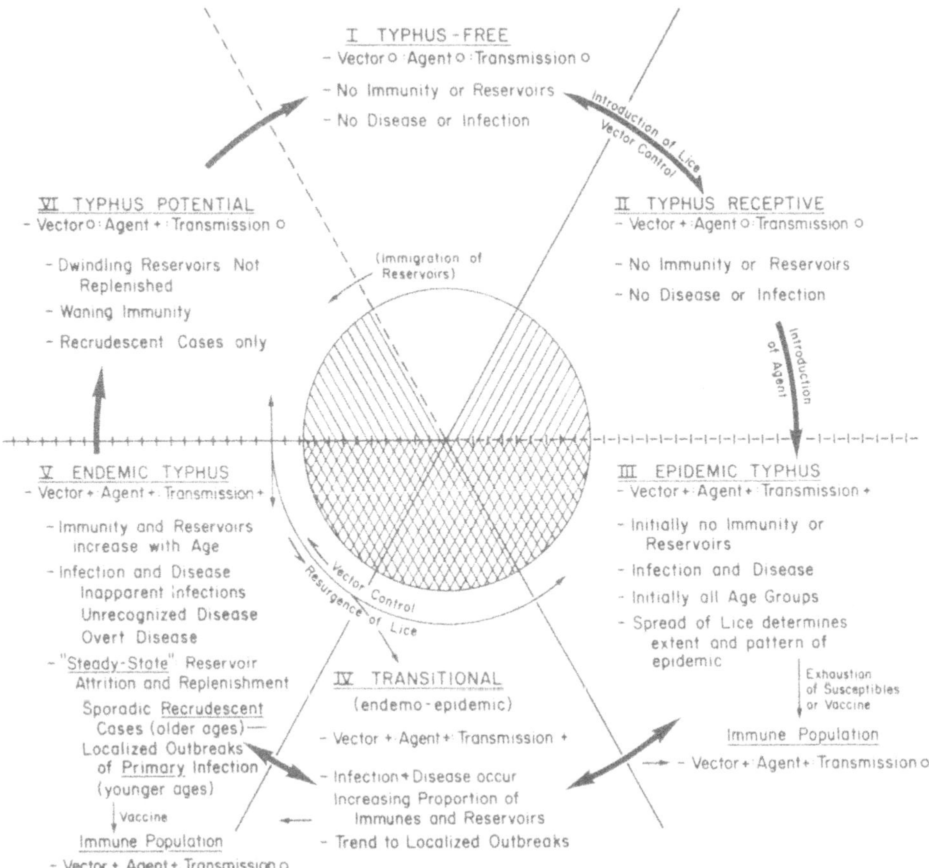

Fig. 1 Diagrammatic representation of the major interactions among the typhus rickettsia, the body louse and human beings in the natural history of louse-borne epidemic typhus fever. Major epidemiological stages are identified by Roman numerals.

eradicating the organism from the human reservoir, where its presence is the key to endemicity; it now cannot be removed except by natural attrition.

Actual examples of all these different stages with complete, fully documented, quantitative data on all the important variables just do not exist. However, the recent history of typhus in Poland, compiled from various sources (9-11) and synthesized into a graphic summary in Figure 2, illustrates many important points. Thus, following the large epidemic during and after World War I, the disease appeared to settle down into an endemo-epidemic pattern, somewhere between Stages IV and V, with a large fraction of the disease follwoing the typical seasonal pattern of louse-borne primary infection, as shown for the years 1936-1939. These cases probably occurred only in certain segments of this large, complex population. No doubt socio-economic compartmentalization of different sub-populations within the whole permitted the preservation of typhus in certain segments side by side with the simultaneous accumulation of large numbers of susceptibles in typhus-free segments. With the disastrous disruptions of World War II, the diaphanous barriers between typhus-bearing and typhus-free segments disintegrated, conditions for widespread lousiness were created in all segments of the population and both vector and agent spread rapidly to produce a massive epidemic, more or less equivalent to Stage III. With the cessation of the war and the return of the population towards a higher standard of living and hygiene, probably aided by the newly discovered insecticides, the incidence of disease diminished and for a time appeared to be settling back into its pre-war endemo-epidemic pattern. In the early 1950's, however, the seasonal variation became less pronounced and the cases were found to consist of two types: (a) recrudescent cases occurring steadily throughout the year in the older age groups who had experienced primary infection years before, and (b) louse-borne primary typhus cases classically in the cold months in the younger age groups who represented the major accumulation of susceptibles. The pattern of typhus had thus shifted into a Stage V or endemic form. Further reduction of the vector with elimination of transmission could easily shift the pattern into Stage VI.

Figure 3 summarizes the age relationship in the endemic situation between immunes, reservoirs and recrudescent typhus cases on the one hand and the susceptibles and primary typhus on the other, which is the mechanism whereby the attrition of older reservoirs through death is offset by the creation of new reservoirs. The figure also shows how either vector control or mass immunization can interfere with this process.

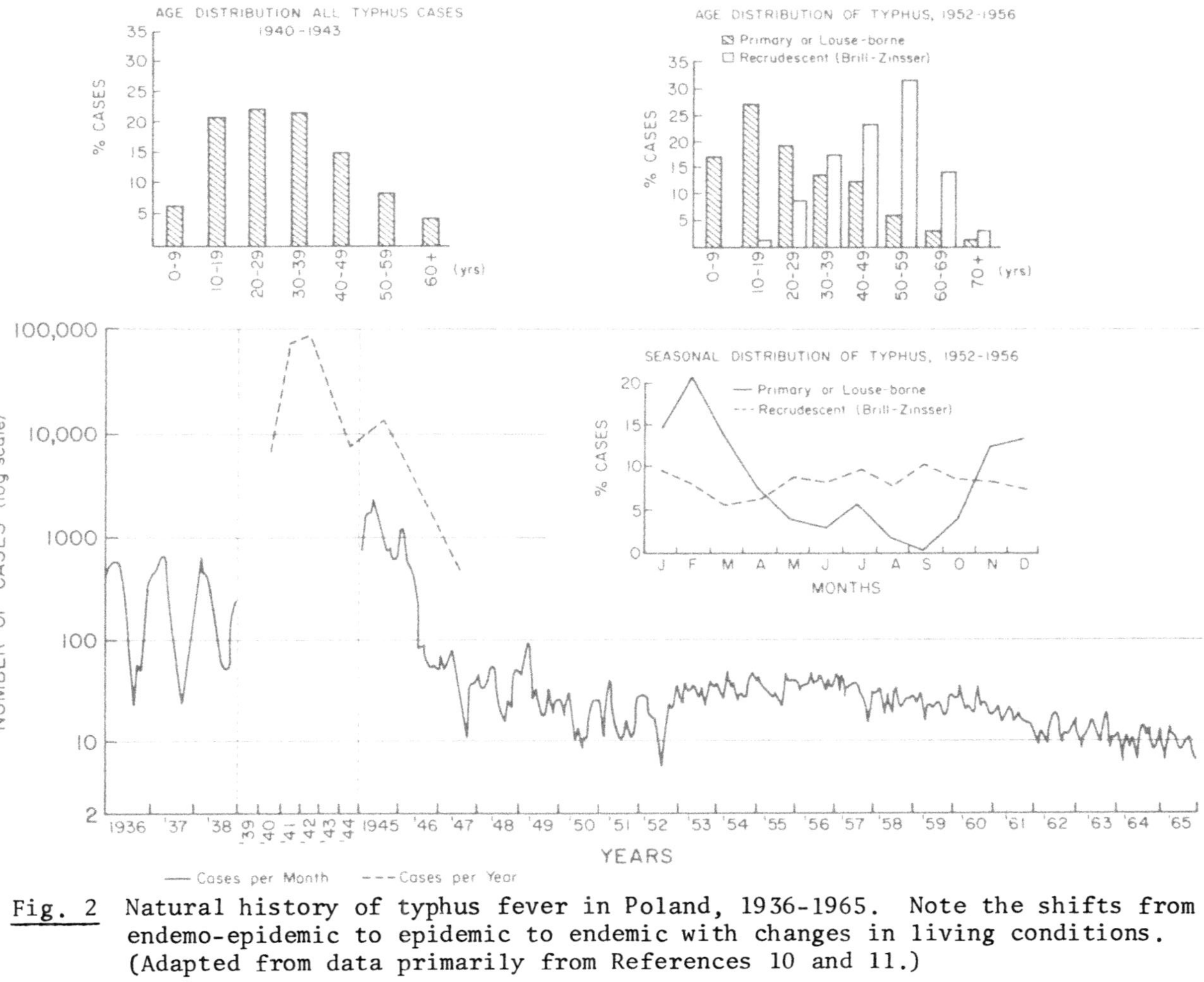

Fig. 2 Natural history of typhus fever in Poland, 1936-1965. Note the shifts from endemo-epidemic to epidemic to endemic with changes in living conditions. (Adapted from data primarily from References 10 and 11.)

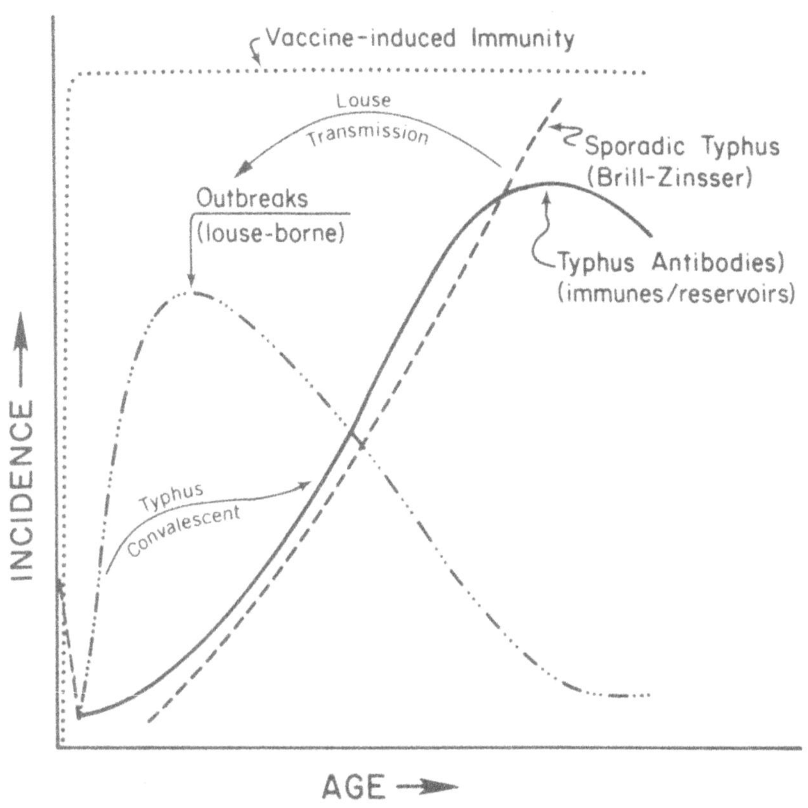

Fig. 3 Schematic representation of endemic state of typhus showing the age distribution (a) of typhus immunes (who are also typhus reservoirs) as revealed by sero-epidemiological studies, (b) of cases of recrudescent typhus derived from "(a)" and (c) of cases of primary louse-borne typhus which replenish the reservoir population which is being depleted by natural attrition, yielding a "steady state" type of equilibrium. Elimination of either the vector or the susceptible segment of the population will alter the dynamics, but in significantly different ways. (Basic patterns of antibody and recrudescent and primary typhus derived from examination of data in References 10-15.)

PRINCIPLES OF TYPHUS CONTROL

In 1937, a Committee of Experts at a conference held under the auspices of the League of Nations (18) summarized the principles of typhus control, based upon the accumulated knowledge and experience at that time (Table 1). In drawing up this list of principles, it would seem that the Committee had in mind primarily the sharp outbreak or epidemic form of the disease typical of the European setting. With minor modifications in details, these principles are still valid for control of the localized outbreak or epidemic. However, additional modifications now seem desirable to define a comprehensive program generally applicable to all epidemiological stages in the natural history of typhus, to large national or regional problems as well as to more localized outbreaks, and to accommodate great variations in logistic aspects and resources. A comprehensive approach must not only be concerned with the urgent immediate problem of disease prevention in any given outbreak but also with the ultimate long-range management of the basic underlying problems if any real impact is to be made on the disease. Table 2 emphasizes the key role that preventing the creation of new reservoirs plays in attaining the ideal or some reasonably acceptable compromise.

Table 3 summarizes some characteristics of the measures currently available for typhus control. It is obvious that none is perfect, but each can be used to advantage under certain conditions.

REALITIES OF THE PROBLEMS OF TYPHUS CONTROL IN DEVELOPING COUNTRIES

In many developing countries, typhus appears to exist in the Stage V of endemicity, if one can rely upon the history, reported cases and scant serological data (19-29). Figure 4, an example taken from the data of Montoya *et al* (19), shows the age distribution of typhus antibodies in 1954 in certain populations in Peru where typhus has been a problem for an untold number of years. It is easy to predict that the pattern of recrudescent and primary cases of typhus, if identified, would conform to that depicted in the preceding Figure 3.

The validity of such an extrapolation from sero-epidemiological data is reinforced by the occurrence of sporadic explosive outbreaks of typhus so common in remote villages of the mountainous regions of the world, such as in Mexico, Central America and South America where there is reason to believe that the sero-epidemiological profile is similar to that just described for Peru (23-29).

TABLE I

GENERAL MEASURES FOR COMBATTING TYPHUS

1937 LON Principles for Epidemic Control	1972 Comprehensive Program
1. Case finding	I. Recognition and Definition of Problem A. Reporting and laboratory diagnosis B. Epidemiological study and classification of problem C. Assessment of logistics and resources D. Selection of appropriate control measures from "B" and "C"
2. Isolation of cases	II. Interruption of Transmission A. Short-term: Immediate effect
3. Isolation of districts and regions	1. Isolation of cases and regions 2. Vector control: Insecticides a. assessment of resistance
4. Delousing	b. delousing (1) Contacts
5. Immunization of individuals and selected groups	(2) Mass program 3. Immunization: Elimination of susceptibles 4. ? Chemoprophylaxis (limited usefullness)
a. Vaccine	B. Long-range: Ultimate eradication
b. Seroprophylaxis	1. Prevention of new reservoir formation a. Eradication of vector (1) ? Insecticides (2) Laundry, bathing, education b. Maintenance of high state of immunity in all age groups 2. Elimination of existing reservoirs a. Natural attrition b. ? Chemotherapy - no rickettsia-cidal agent yet available
	III. Treatment of cases A. Reduction of morbidity and mortality B. Reduction of period of infectivity for louse C. Prevention of reservoir state (not yet possible)

TABLE II

OBJECTIVES OF TYPHUS CONTROL MEASURES

1. Immediate: Stop disease
2. Intermediate: Prevent creation of new reservoirs of agent
3. Long-range Ideal: Eradication of agent and vector

TABLE III

CHARACTERISTICS OF AVAILABLE TYPHUS CONTROL MEASURES

1. Louse Control
    a. Prevents disease
    b. Interrupts transmission, even if lice are not eradicated
    c. Eradication difficult; effect often transient; resistance may interfere
    d. Prevents creation of new typhus reservoirs
    e. Uninfected population remains receptive to re-introduction of agent
2. Immunization (ideal)
    a. Prevents disease
    b. Interrupts transmission
    c. Prevents creation of new reservoirs
    d. Population unreceptive to re-introduction of agent even if vector is not eliminated
3. Chemotherapy-Chemoprophylaxis (present status)
    a. Probably can prevent disease, but not infection
    b. Shortens period of transmissibility to lice
    c. Probably does not prevent creation of new reservoirs
    d. Reduces morbidity and mortality of established cases

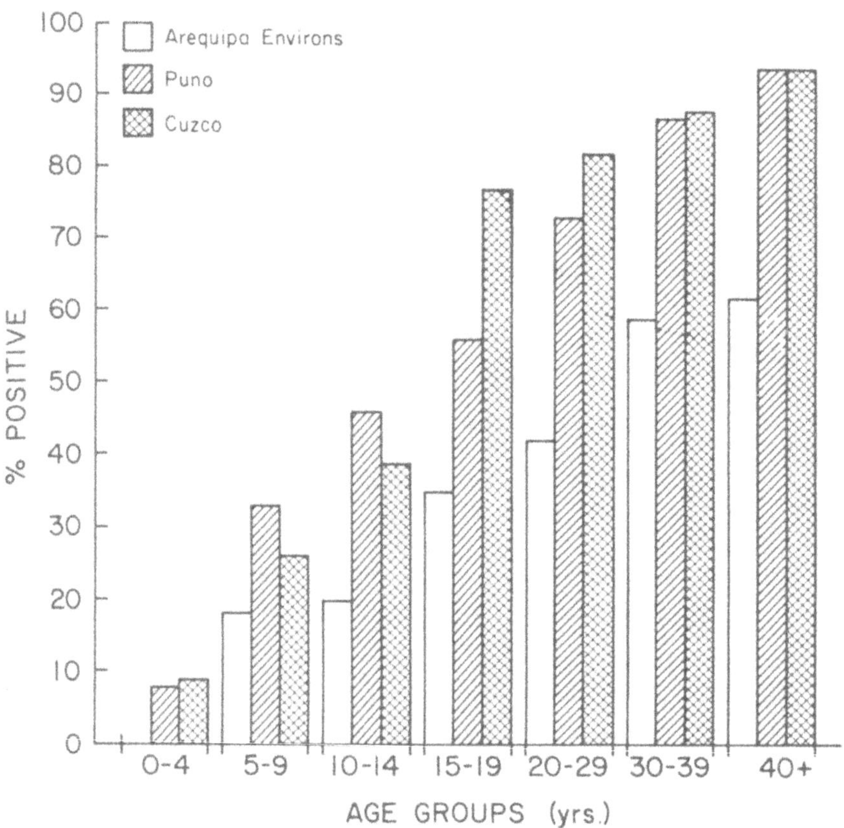

(adapted from data in Montoya *et al*, 1955)

Fig. 4 Age distribution for typhus antibodies in three typhus-endemic localities in Peru in 1954 (adapted from data in Reference 19). Considered as reservoirs, it would be predicted that these typhus convalescents should give rise to a substantial number of recrudescences followed by louse-borne primary infections. Very limited data on age distribution of reported typhus (27) suggest that this does occur but there has been no differentiation between recrudescent and primary cases. Moreover, there is serologic evidence from the same region (64) for the occurrence of between 13 and 51 infections for every recognized case over a 3 1/2 year period of surveillance.

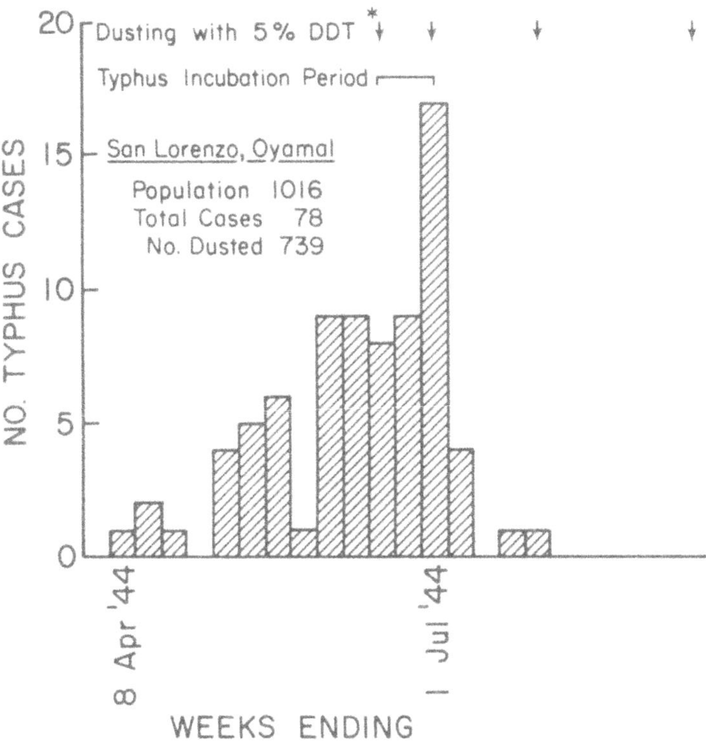

Fig. 5 A typical village outbreak of typhus in an endemic region. Had this outbreak not been controlled with DDT, it would have been expected to follow a natural course typical of village outbreaks in this region in which the declining phase resembles the build-up roughly in shape and time scale. (Adapted from Reference 25.)

The classical story of recognized typhus, repeated so many times over the years in different places where the disease is endemic, is that word is received by health authorities of a local outbreak of serious disease with some deaths which resembles typhus, often in some remote place. A health team is sent out to investigate and control the outbreak. By the time the team reaches the site, after the usual delays imposed by problems of travel, etc., additional cases have occurred. Patients with disease are treated and the population is dusted with insecticides one or more times over a short period, often without knowing whether or not the lice in that locality are indeed susceptible to the insecticide(s) being used. Perhaps even some killed vaccine is administered. The outbreak ceases, as a result either of the control measures or of the seasonal pattern.

However, there is growing evidence that many more typhus infections actually occur in these areas than are recognized and reported (9,64). The sporadic case of recrudescent or primary typhus, occurring on a background of other similar febrile illnesses, is not recognized and inapparent infections also seem to occur. The typical localized outbreak just described is then merely the tip of the iceberg of typhus that is visible while the bulk of the transmission and infection remains unrecognized. Thus, the practice of limiting the attack on typhus to these sporadic outbreaks of overt disease as they occur has in fact several serious disadvantages: (a) it does not recognize most typhus infections which are occurring; (b) it recognizes typhus only when many people have become seriously ill and some have died; (c) new typhus reservoirs have been created; (d) the vector is not eradicated and indeed insecticide resistance may be enhanced; and (e) no permanent or significant change has been made in the basic epidemiological climate or future typhus potential.

Some of the main factors which contribute to typhus endemicity and interfere with optimal application of control measures in developing countries fall into the following categories:

1. Living conditions which are conducive to chronic, endemic lousiness, possibly enhanced by cultural factors related to lousiness.

2. Difficult communications, both in regard to notifying health authorities about disease occurrence and accessibility of population for prompt and repeated application of control measures.

3. Limited resources: economic, trained man-power, transport, etc.

4. Poorly developed systems for reporting disease and inadequate laboratory diagnostic facilities.

5. Political: hostility of population segments towards representatives of central government; rejection of government-sponsored programs (30).

6. Control measures and concepts based on experience with unusual acute, transient situations in advanced countries are applied directly, and sometimes inappropriately, to the chronic, persisting conditions in the less well-developed, emergent countries.

Though not exhaustive, this list identifies some of the factors which may influence the choice and efficacy of control measures in any given situation.

APPLICATION OF SPECIFIC CONTROL MEASURES TO TYPHUS PROBLEMS IN DEVELOPING COUNTRIES

Vector Control Through Application of Insecticides

Because of the early dramatic successes in the control of typhus by the mass application of insecticides in Europe during and immediately after World War II (25-28), great reliance has been placed on this measure for control of typhus (35). However, this approach has not always met with such success in some of the less well-developed areas of the world for the reason that inadequate attention has been paid to the basic epidemiological, ecological and biological factors, to the enormous logistic problems and to the limitations in resources.

In retrospect, the situations in which insecticides have had their greatest effect on the long-term control of typhus differed significantly from the conditions existing in most areas with current persisting typhus problems. For example, the dramatic effect on the 1943-44 typhus epidemic in Naples was probably not only due to the powerful action of DDT on the louse (33) but also to the fact that the conditions contributing to lousiness were transient; summer was approaching and there was a relatively rapid return towards the former higher standard of living and hygiene, which then held lousiness at a reduced level without continued intense insecticide application. Moreover, DDT dusting was accomplished efficiently and rapidly through the enormous logistic potential and resources of an organized military force.

In sharp contrast, the conditions conducive to lousiness, and lousiness itself, in less well-developed countries where typhus is a problem, are not transient, but tend to be long-standing, persistent and chronically endemic - almost a way of life. When an insecticide is applied once, or perhaps even a few times over a short period of time in this setting, there may be a prompt initial, but evanescent, reduction in lousiness (27, 31-34); but after a short time the incidence of lousiness may again approach its former level (27), as shown in Figure 6. Thus, to achieve long-term vector control without basic changes in the way of life, a vigorous program of indefinite duration, consisting of repeated insecticide application at appropriate intervals, must be maintained, unless complete eradication can be achieved without subsequent re-infestation. This may be logistically impractical or even biologically unsound.

Despite these limitations, insecticides have had dramatic effects on the small localized outbreaks of typhus which characterize the endemic or endemo-epidemic situations, as shown in Figure 7. Thus, a single or a few applications of insecticide over a short period of time can reduce lousiness to a sufficiently low level that the transmission chain of typhus is broken and the outbreak ceases, even though the louse population may subsequently return to its former level and the basic epidemiological state is unchanged.

However, when insecticides are used suboptimally in the face of endemic lousiness, the lice may develop resistance to the insecticide (35). Figure 8 illustrates another localized explosive typhus outbreak in a Mexican village, typical of the endemic situation, about two decades after the initial introduction of DDT into Mexico; a little over a decade after institution of a nation-wide campaign to eradicate the body louse; and about five years after DDT-resistant lice were first recognized in Mexico. In contrast to the sharp effect of DDT in the previously described outbreak, there is really no discernible effect of mass dusting with DDT in this instance. The disease continued to follow the expected seasonal pattern of an uncontrolled outbreak in this setting. Although data are not available for this village, one can only assume that the lice had become resistant to DDT.

Today DDT-resistance is common among body lice in many parts of the world, resistance to lindane (gamma-hexachlorohexane) is being reported with increasing frequency (35), and a high degree of resistance to malathion has been found in Burundi (36).

These are a few examples of the problems being encountered in attempts to control the typhus vector with insecticides in endemic situations. Other approaches to louse control, too extensive to consider here, are possible and are probably feasible under these circumstances.

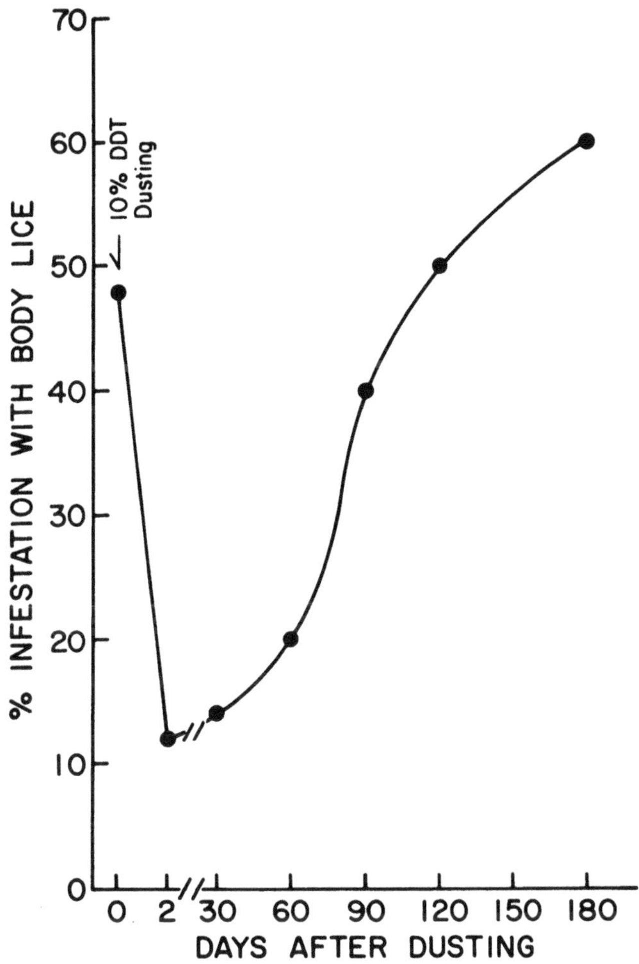

Fig. 6 Effect of a single DDT dusting on the incidence of lousiness in a Peruvian village in a typhus-endemic zone (adapted from Reference 27). Note the rapid and dramatic - but not complete - reduction in the incidence of lousiness after dusting, followed by the gradual rise. Quantitative data of this kind collected over such a long period of time are rare in the literature. Though inadequate to eradicate lice, an effect of this kind may interrupt the transmission cycle of typhus in typical village outbreaks.

MEXICO: CONTROL OF TYPHUS OUTBREAK IN A VILLAGE WITH DDT

(adapted from Ortiz-Mariott et al, 1944, 1945)

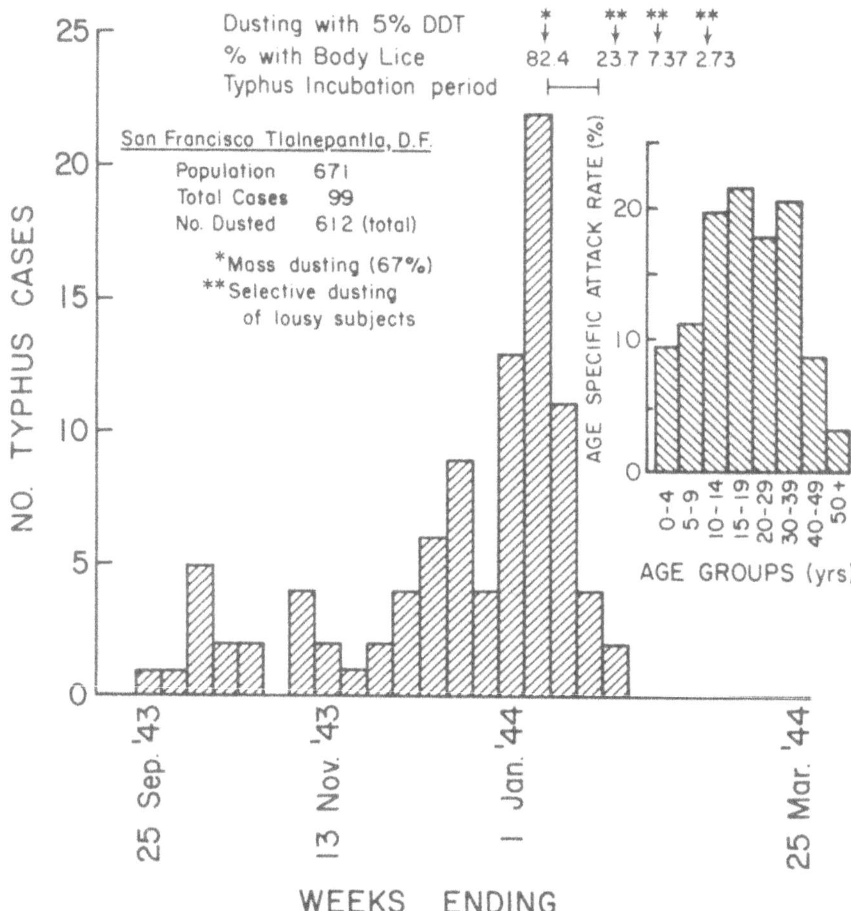

Fig. 7 Control of a typical village typhus outbreak in an endemic zone with repeated applications of DDT (adapted and interpreted from data in References 25 and 26). Note the typical age distribution of cases and the significant - but not complete - reduction in lousiness, which would be expected to rise again, as demonstrated in Figure 6. In the outbreaks illustrated here and in Figure 5, there was a marked reduction in incidence of typhus cases within one incubation period of typhus after the first application of DDT.

WINTER TYPHUS OUTBREAK IN MEXICAN MOUNTAIN VILLAGE: POOR RESPONSE TO MASS DDT DUSTING-? UNRECOGNIZED RESISTANCE.* (Compiled from Olivero Toro and Ortiz Mariotte, 1964)

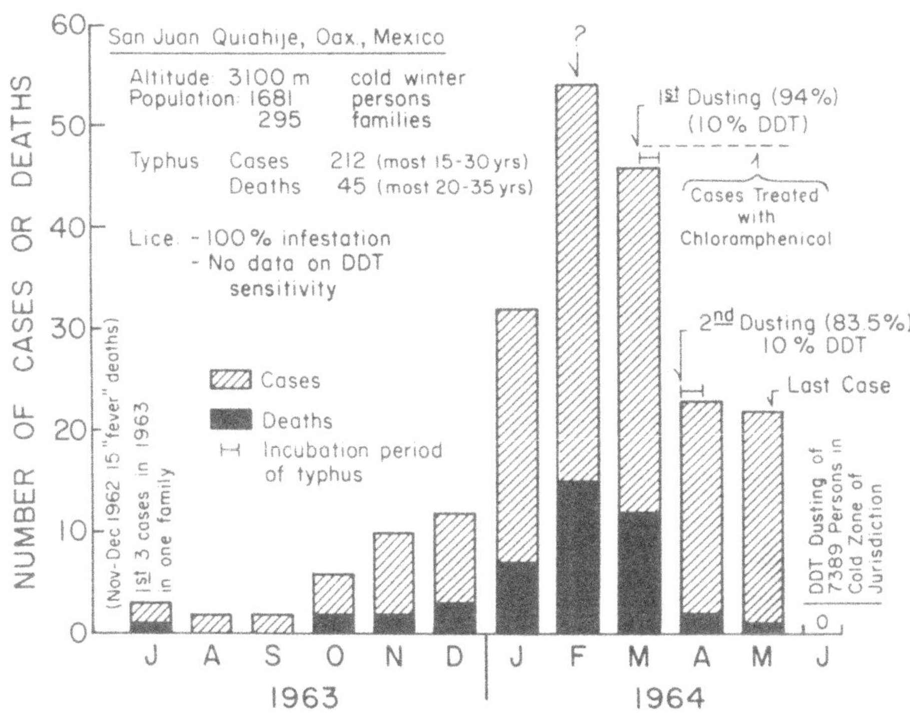

*DDT resistance in body lice first reported from Mexico in 1959 (WHO)

Fig. 8 Failure of DDT to alter the course of a village typhus outbreak, probably because of unrecognized DDT-resistance among body lice. Note that (a) the time increments here are months, instead of weeks as in Figures 5 and 7, (b) there was little recognizable effect of dusting within an average typhus incubation period and (c) the course of this outbreak is very similar to that of untreated village outbreaks. (Assembled, adapted and re-interpreted from Reference 23).

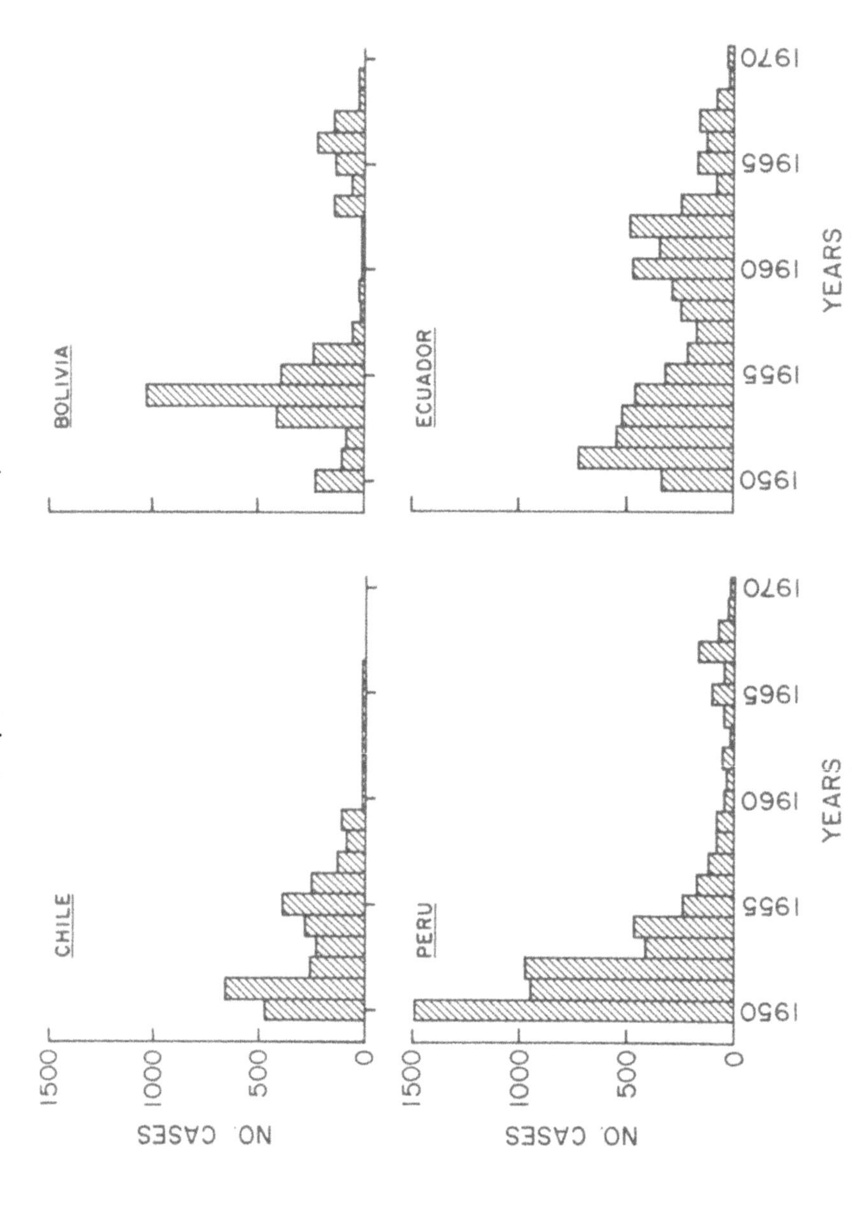

Fig. 9 Reported cases of typhus (1950-1970) in four Andean countries where typhus has been endemic.

Despite the gloomy picture presented above, louse control through insecticides is an important component of typhus control and when used appropriately can accomplish: (a) a transient effect sufficient to stop small localized outbreaks of disease, even though the vector is not eradicated and conditions conducive to lousiness persist; (b) eradication of lice in small populations not subject to re-infestation; and (c) acceleration of the disappearance of lice when basic living conditions are improving. However, it is questionable if insecticides alone can eradicate or even produce long-term control in the vast, relatively inaccessible populations of depressed areas where conditions conducive to lousiness remain unchanged. Nevertheless. there has in fact been a gradual decline in reported cases of typhus from several countries which have instituted some kind of louse-control program (27-29), as is illustrated in Figure 9. The explanations for this, however, may be complex, including a possible rise in standard of living, health education and other factors, and may not be entirely the result of the insecticide programs.

Elimination of the Typhus-Susceptible Segment of the Human Population Through Active Immunization

Immunity following typhus fever is usually strong and long-lasting; naturally occurring antigenic shifts in *R. prowazeki* have not been proven. Since even the immunity following natural typhus fever is non-sterile, i.e., the organism persists, it is unknown if even the best possible vaccine would prevent a vaccinated person, on subsequent exposure to a virulent strain, from acquiring and harboring that strain, thus becoming a potential reservoir. At the opposite extreme, neither is it known if vaccine given to typhus convalescents, i.e., reservoirs, would prevent recrudescence of infection. Nevertheless, immunization with a good vaccine could be expected: (a) to prevent disease in the individual; (b) to prevent transmission, and hence reservoir creation, in the immunized population even if the louse persists; and (c) to protect lousy typhus-receptive populations against introduction of the agent. Immunization of the majority of a population would thus divert it from subjection to the usual epidemiological sequence and into a special category. And if a high level of immunity were maintained for a sufficiently long period of time, natural attrition of reservoirs could proceed in the presence of lice without the risk of outbreaks of primary infection.

Realization of these ideal objectives depends upon (a) the capacity to produce an acceptable safe vaccine which will induce the desired degree and duration of immunity and (b) the feasibility of administering it to a population according to the regimen required for effectiveness.

Variations of two general types of typhus vaccine, (a) killed and (b) living, were explored from the earliest days (2,37). For the most part, however, yolk sac-grown, killed vaccines were used by the American, Canadian and British Forces in World War II (38) and have been used by many countries for both civilians and the military since then. These vaccines, unfortunately, are still subject to many problems of production, antigen content, potency and assay, recently reviewed in other reports (39,40). Aside from very limited vaccination-challenge studies, which suggested that some, but not complete, protection was afforded by certain vaccines (41, 42,57,59), no large-scale adequately controlled trials have been carried out successfully so as to provide the necessary quantitative data on effectiveness. Moreover, the combined experience of the Allied military forces with killed typhus vaccines in World War II did not yield satisfactory information on the degree of protection afforded against acquiring typhus fever even though it clearly indicated that the vaccines modified the disease and prevented deaths in persons who developed typhus after having received one or more doses of vaccine (43-47,65,66). In addition, the infectivity for lice of patients with vaccine-modified disease was found to be reduced but not eliminated (48-51). These considerations, along with the requirement for multiple doses and frequent boosters, suggest that currently available killed vaccines may not be adequate to achieve the potential benefits of immunization mentioned above, especially with regard to changing the basic epidemiologic status.

With the recognition of a spontaneous attenuated mutant of *R. prowazeki*, the Madrid E strain, by Clavero and Perez Gallardo (52,53), a new candidate for a living attenuated vaccine was introduced. Fox and his associates (54-64) explored its potential as a vaccine in a series of comprehensive studies from the laboratory, through vaccination-challenge studies in human volunteers, to a large-scale field trial in Peru in the 1950's. Most significantly, from the standpoint of typhus control programs, as we have presented the problem here, was the fact that a single inoculation of the living attenuated E strain produced a strong immunity to virulent epidemic typhus challenge which lasted for at least five years. Two types of reaction to the vaccine were encountered: (a) a dose-dependent early reaction (24-48 hrs) which could be eliminated by adjustment of dosage and (b) a late reaction in up to 14 percent of the people, 9-14 days after vaccination, which varied from mild malaise and headache to a brief highly modified febrile illness which never required treatment. These reactions, however, did not interfere with the acceptability of the vaccine in the field trial in Peru which involved over 30,000 people. Other groups have since investigated the E strain to greater or lesser degrees (65-78), with somewhat variable conclusions regarding the importance of reactions as regards acceptability (see next section).

TABLE IV

COMPARISON OF KILLED AND LIVING ATTENUATED TYPHUS VACCINES

Category	Characteristic of	
	Killed Vaccines	E Strain Vaccine
1. No. of Doses	Multiple; timing important	1
2. Time for Effect	Relatively long for optimum	Prob. 7-10 days
3. Duration of Immunity	? Short, requiring periodic boosters. Good booster after many years	$\geq$ 5 yrs
4. Protection		
a. Clinical Disease	Incomplete but modifies	Strong
b. Rickettsemia	Incomplete but reduces	Prob. none
c. Louse Infection	Incomplete but reduces	Prob. none
d. Reservoir Creation	Incomplete prevention	Unknown
e. Recrudescence		Unknown
5. Reactions	1) Local and systemic "endotoxin" reactions with potent vaccines	1) Early dose dependent in both immunes and non-immunes
	2) Local and systemic delayed type hypersensitivity	2) Late reactions--modified disease in non-immunes
	3) ? Immediate allergy to host cell components	
6. Problems	1) Protective antigen(s) not known	? Reversion to virulence
	2) Potency and potency assay	

The E strain has been under study at the University of Maryland for well over a decade and a comprehensive account of these studies is being prepared for publication (79). Experience with its use as a vaccine is being accumulated in a step-wise manner in military populations in the U.S.A. and in different epidemiologic situations with regard to typhus control in developing countries. Although these studies are still in progress and observations are still being made, some of the results available to date, summarized very briefly below, would appear to have some bearing on the problems of typhus control in developing countries.

The first study to be described is a controlled field trial of the E strain vaccine during a large-scale typhus epidemic in Burundi. The sequence of events leading to the occurrence of typhus on an epidemic scale, essentially equivalent to Stage III, in Burundi is complex and is being documented and analyzed elsewhere (36,80, 81). Suffice it to say here that a very large susceptible population, including all age groups, had built up throughout the country, that body lice had become highly resistant to DDT over much of the country and to malathion over extensive but lesser areas and that lousiness was essentially universal throughout the highland regions. A major spread of typhus began in the early 1960's and rose to a very high level of epidemic activity in many parts of the country by 1967-1969, when our studies were initiated. The dispersion of the indigenous population over the land probably influenced the rate and pattern of spread. At the present time, the disease is probably entering the transitional or endemo-epidemic Stage IV of typhus in parts of the country. For all of the reasons previously mentioned, it was not possible for government health authorities to mount an effective louse control program for the entire country, although some success was achieved with lindane-containing powders in isolated instances of accessible populations concentrated in refugee camps.

After identifying the epidemic as louse-borne typhus in 1967 and making some preliminary observations on its epidemiology, a controlled field trial of the attenuated living E strain vaccine was proposed, accepted, planned and finally initiated in 1969. Ten hills in the communes of Katara and Matongo, determined by inspection to be one of the most densely populated and active typhus areas at that time, were selected for the project.

Although the local conditions might impress the casual observer as being too primitive to permit controlled study, closer observation would reveal that all the components for a sophisticated study were in fact present: (a) a large epidemic of typhus in progress; (b) a stable, dense (500-600/sq. mile) population, extraordinarily sophisticated in the recognition of the various clinical types of typhus, who feared the disease, greatly desired help, were extremely cooperative, and who could be identified through the tax-book required to be carried by the head of every household; (c) a sophisticated local civil organization with interested and conscientious local administrators at the commune and colline level, who participated actively and enthusiastically in all phases of the project and whose help with local customs was invaluable; (d) an excellent local communication system, with roads to each colline and drums to spread the word; and (e) a single medical facility, a mission hospital-dispensary, where all illnesses from the region received treatment. Indeed, it would be difficult to find a better-suited local organization and situation anywhere for a study of this kind.

In June and July 1969, 11,164 persons above about one year of age (about 80 percent of the population estimated from census data) were vaccinated by jet gun with a single dose of either Tetanus-Diphtheria toxoid (5,590 persons) or $10^{5.5}EID_{50}$ of the E Strain Vaccine (5,574 persons). People from each hill were directed into the line for one or the other vaccine as they came. A punch-card bearing pertinent data was prepared for each vaccinee. The two groups were remarkably comparable with regard to age, sex distribution and history of previous typhus. The centrally located Katara Mission Dispensary served as headquarters for the study and was the only medical facility in the region where treatment could be received. Numbered study identification cards of the same color as the Dispensary cards were issued to each vaccinee. An intensive surveillance program was instituted for the first 11 weeks following vaccination consisting of a daily ambulance service to each hill to transport <u>any</u> sick person and house-to-house visits (each house was numbered) by health workers and team members every seven to ten days with the help of the local "notables". After the first 11 weeks, when the team from the U.S. left and the pattern had been established with the population for prompt free treatment at the dispensary, modified surveillance was instituted in which all patients presenting at the dispensary were screened and managed, as during the intensive surveillance, by a single, highly interested Belgian Sister who had become extraordinarily competent in this program. Serum specimens were obtained from a sample of the population at the time of vaccination and again six weeks later. Each ill person had at least paired serum specimens drawn, had a detailed clinical record maintained and was given appropriate treatment.

The pre-vaccination distribution of antibodies was comparable in both control and E strain groups. Six weeks after vaccination a marked shift in antibody pattern was found in the E strain group, with only two of 181 individuals in the sample failing to show complement fixing antibody conversion whereas the antibody pattern of the control group was essentially unchanged. Thus, as judged by antibody response, the E strain vaccine accomplished what it theoretically should have done, i.e., changed the basic epidemiological climate and removed the population from the expected natural epidemiological sequence, as shown previously in Figure 1.

Surveillance for typhus cases showed that this was indeed the case as far as prevention of disease is concerned. In the first 11 weeks of intensive surveillance 25 cases of laboratory-confirmed typhus occurred in the control groups whereas none occurred in the E strain group. And at the end of 14 months, which included about 11 months of modified surveillance, 49 cases of confirmed typhus occurred in the control group and three cases in the E strain group, a protection rate of 94 percent. We are now assessing the effect over the second year of modified surveillance.

The E strain vaccine has shown its capacity to protect against disease in the face of an epidemic. If a sufficient proportion of a population were vaccinated, these data suggest that transmission would promptly cease and the creation of new reservoirs would stop, even without a change in the incidence of lousiness. This could have been done throughout Burundi if the vaccine had been given on a mass saturation scale, but vaccination programs of this kind must progress in a step-wise manner to prevent unexpected catastrophes and to gain sufficient experience and confidence. In the meantime, however, an enormous typhus reservoir has been created and the disease, now entering the transitional Stage IV will likely proceed to a stable endemic Stage V which will be difficult to manage by vector control alone, unless there is a very dramatic improvement in the capacity of the country as well as its neighbors to <u>mount</u> and <u>maintain</u> a truly effective country-wide louse control program.

Another field study of the E strain vaccine was initiated last year in Bolivia where typhus has been endemic, probably for centuries. The overt disease pattern here has been one of isolated and localized, sporadic outbreaks of typhus, typical of the highly endemic Stage V. Three widely separated populations, totalling about 8,000 people and representative of the typhus situation on the Bolivian altiplano, were selected for study. Because the efficacy of the E strain vaccine in an epidemic in Burundi in a controlled trial had been demonstrated and because of logistic problems related to resources and accessibility of populations, the plan in Bolivia was (a) to study the epidemiology of typhus in these areas, (b) to vaccinate the total populations in each area, if possible, (c) to assess acceptability insofar as possible, (d) to measure the antibody conversion and persistence patterns and (e) to assess the impact of the vaccine on this endemic situation by whatever means might be possible. This study is still in its early stages. However, it was possible to obtain pre-vaccination serum specimens from over 16 percent of these populations and to vaccinate nearly 60 percent down to about one year of age without incident. Six-week post-vaccination serum specimens have been collected but testing is not yet complete.

The age-specific CF antibody distribution in the pre-vaccination sera from all three areas showed a definite but low incidence in the very young, progressing steadily to an incidence of between 60 and 70 percent of people in the 50-59-year age group. The age distribution of antibodies is typical of the endemic Stage V. Though the data are not available, it is obvious that recrudescent typhus must be occurring in these older people and that louse-born transmission is taking place, often to the young if this degree of endemicity is to be maintained. It is also obvious that, if this pattern is representative of the situation throughout the altiplano, an enormous number of unrecognized infections must be taking place. Only the sharp localized outbreaks involving numbers of people are now recognized, i.e., just the tip of the iceberg previously mentioned. We are hopeful that the E strain vaccine will change the basic epidemiological climate here as well and will prevent the creation of new reservoirs as now must be occurring through inapparent, unrecognized or overt infections. To do so, however, the young must be included in the vaccination program, for these form the bulk of the susceptibles who now maintain the louse-borne transmission phase of the disease. It is of interest, but not significant with regard to assessing the protective action of the E strain vaccine, that a typical sharp outbreak of typhus with 31 cases and seven deaths has been recognized recently in a village near one of our study populations. We hope to be able to continue these studies on a quantitative basis in order to assess the validity of our concepts and the usefulness of the E strain vaccine.

PROBLEMS OF THE E STRAIN VACCINE

From the very beginning of studies on the E strain as a vaccine for man, as with any other living vaccine, investigators have been concerned with: (a) reactions in persons receiving the vaccine, i.e., acceptability; (b) potential for unrestricted growth in the person whose defense mechanisms have been compromised; and (c) stability of the state of attenuation, both in regard to possible increase in virulence which might place both individual and community at risk as well as possible decrease in virulence resulting in loss of immunogenicity. These are discussed separately below.

Reactions to E Strain Vaccine

As with all vaccines and especially with living vaccines, the matter of reactions looms large in importance as regards acceptability and usefulness. Since few vaccines are completely devoid of any reactions whatsoever, the suitability of vaccines are often judged on the basis of the frequency and severity of reactions relative to the need for, and benefits expected from, a given vaccine under a given set of circumstances. For example, smallpox vaccine is not without reactions and even severe risks, but there is no hesitancy to use it when smallpox is a real threat. Indeed, in the past, deliberate inoculation with virulent variola virus was accepted by some as preferable to naturally acquired disease. In many countries now, however, the threat of smallpox is so small that even the risks entailed with the use of vaccinia virus vaccine are considered too great. In the same way, the relative merits of the E strain vaccine should be considered against the typhus disease problem in any given situation.

The unique immunogenicity of the E strain undoubtedly rests upon its capacity to induce an attenuated but immunizing infection in man (54-79). Indeed, administration of chloramphenicol to personse inoculated with E strain suppresses the antibody response (79). However, it has not been possible to isolate the E strain from vaccinated human subjects, either by the inoculation of eggs with blood or by the feeding of lice on such subjects (55,64,82).

On careful observation, two kinds of clinical responses, i.e., reactions, have been recognized following inoculation of human subjects (54-79).

(a) An early reaction, both local and systemic, in the first two to three days after inoculation. This early reaction is dose dependent and can be avoided by reducing the dose, within limits, without significantly depressing its immunogenicity. It occurs in both non-immune and immune subjects.

(b) A late reaction, usually 9-14 days after inoculation and considered by most as an expression of attenuated infection. It is not influenced greatly by dose and is suppressed in immune subjects. Some manifestations of the late reaction have been observed in up to about 14 percent of non-immune subjects. Its severity ranges from simple malaise and mild headache to a modified typhus characterized by fever, headache, malaise and occasionally a rash in a small proportion of subjects. Even the most severe reactions resolve without specific therapy but apparently may be shortened by antibiotics. There is some suggestion that, like typhus itself, these late reactions are more severe in middle-aged persons than in the younger age groups.

The late reaction is the one of concern regarding acceptability of the E strain as a vaccine. Judgements regarding the relative importance of these reactions must be made on the basis of the morbidity it produces under the different conditions of use. Thus, Fox and his co-workers (63,64) found that the E strain vaccine was generally well tolerated in a large field trial in a typhus-endemic area in Peru. Our own studies in the U.S.A. in over 1,000 military recruits in the 18-20-year age group revealed that the E strain was as well tolerated as the killed vaccine, as judged by interference with duty (79). Russian investigators (65-75) found the reactions tolerable in their early experience with the E strain but became somewhat more concerned about them as the numbers of inoculated persons increased. Indeed, they have more recently investigated, with some success, the possibility of giving both killed and living attenuated vaccines simultaneously to suppress the late reactions. Egyptian investigators (76,77) reported that the incidence and severity of reactions were tolerable and did not affect the daily activity of 1,350 persons vaccinated in a village near Cairo. Finally, we have found that the E strain vaccine was acceptable to the populations in our recent field trials in both Burundi and Bolivia. More information of this kind is needed. However, the growing experience is that the E strain vaccine is well tolerated by populations in typhus zones; and the reactions experienced are indeed minor compared with full-blown typhus fever.

Potential for Unrestricted Multiplication in the Person Whose Defense Mechanisms Have Been Compromised

It is possible that an agent which behaves as an attenuated strain in normal healthy subjects might behave as a virulent strain in the subject whose defense mechanisms have been compromised by genetic defect, acquired disease or physical and chemical agents. Only a limited number of animal studies bearing on this possibility have been performed with the E strain. Thus Genig (83), comparing the virulent Breinl and the attenuated E strains in guinea pigs which had been stressed with cortisone, found a definite intensification of infection caused by either large or small doses of the virulent Breinl strain but could demonstrate only slight intensification of infection even with very large doses of the E strain and no effect with small doses. Weiss and Dressler (84) found that heavy irradiation of chick embryo entodermal cells in cell culture did not enhance infection with the E strain, but simply elicited a more rapid release of the microorganisms during the period in which the host cells lysed. Fabrikant (79,85) failed to find evidence for enhanced infection with the E strain in both mice and guinea pigs which had been subjected to very heavy doses of whole body X-irradiation. Thus, the limited evidence available to date does not suggest that the E strain readily exhibits dangerous properties in the host whose defenses have been compromised by these two mechanisms.

Stability of Attenuation

The properties of most microorganisms can be altered by manipulation of the selective pressures to which they are exposed. In the case of living attenuated vaccines, the important question is whether or not important changes in properties, i.e., reversion to virulence or the acquisition of new undesirable properties on the one hand or loss of immunogenic capacity on the other, are likely to take place under the conditions of production and use as a vaccine.

When the information available today about the E strain is examined from this point of view, one finds that its properties are remarkably stable under the conditions of production and use as a vaccine. Thus, the vaccine is produced by most investigators by growth in the yolk sac of embryonated hens' eggs. It is the opinion of all the investigators whose work has been reviewed (54-79,86,87) that serial passage in the yolk sac, which now has attained upwards of 270-500 passages, neither enhances nor diminishes its virulence. Indeed, in this host it has displayed a most remarkable stability of attenuation.

When one examines the information that is available about stability of attenuation under conditions of use as a vaccine in man, one finds similar evidence of stability. Although the evidence presented above suggests that the E strain rarely, if ever, causes sufficient rickettsiemia in man to infect lice, several investigators have studied the behavior of the E strain in human body lice. The E strain has been found to grow in the gut epithelium of artificially inoculated lice, but the degree of involvement of the louse gut epithelium has been reported to be lower and the destructive changes less prominent than in the case of infection with a virulent strain (57,82,88,89). Three different investigators have studied the effect of serial louse passage (1-25 serial passages) on the virulence of the E strain and have found no change in the state of its attenuation (82,89,94). Thus, under conditions of use as a vaccine, it would seem highly unlikely that lice would become infected with the E strain but, even if the rare louse did become infected and transmit the strain, it is not likely that this passage through the louse would be accompanied by an increase in virulence.

One possible situation has not been investigated, although there is no evidence yet for its occurrence. It is conceivable that in the rare instance there could be reversion to virulence within the vaccinated human subject. If this did occur, it would not be likely to cause any immediate threat, either to the vaccinated individual or to the community, because (a) such a reversion would presumably occur only in a very small fraction of the organisms present and (b) immunity induced by the attenuated organism develops so rapidly that the hypothetical virulent mutant would have little chance to multiply sufficiently to cause serious disease in the vaccinated person or to infect lice. The possibility, however, that such hypothetical virulent organisms persisting in the vaccinated subject might constitute a reservoir for future recrudescence cannot categorically be excluded at this time and warrants investigation.

When viewed from the perspective of production and use of the E strain as a vaccine for man, the interesting and important, but not entirely surprising, finding of Balayeva (90-93) that a virulent strain, stable in subsequent egg passage, can be selected from the E strain on serial passages in the lungs of mice loses much of its significance as a deterrent to the use of E strain as a vaccine because in practice such an artificial selective pressure would not occur. Of somewhat greater concern, however, is the report by this same group (91) that virulent strains were isolated after one to a few passages in guinea pigs after heavy inoculation with the E strain. There are certain inconsistencies in this report, viz., the reference to fever persisting as long as five days after E strain - a phenomenon unknown in our laboratory - which make it mandatory that these studies be repeated independently in other laboratories where no virulent strains exist and that additional modern genetic techniques be applied to the study and quantitation of variation in virulence in the E strain.

SUMMARY

A. A simplified conceptual framework of the natural history of typhus, based upon the interactions of agent, vector and human host, has been presented with which it is possible (a) to classify most naturally-occurring typhus through measurements which are readily performed with available methods and (b) to predict the effects of control measures and other factors on the basic epidemiological state.

B. The crucial role of the typhus reservoir, i.e., the typhus convalescent person who still harbors the organism and who may subsequently succumb to recrudescent disease in which the rickettsiae again become accessible to lice, has been stressed as it relates the epidemiology of typhus and to the long-range objectives in typhus control.

C. The special problems related to typhus and typhus control in developing countries -- epidemiological, situational and operational -- have been reviewed briefly.

D. The principles of typhus control and the control measures available have been reviewed, in the context of the epidemiological model of the natural history of typhus infections, with regard to (a) their immediate effects on the occurrence of typhus and their capacity to effect a long-range change in the basic epidemiological climate, (b) their practical applicability to typhus control programs in developing countries and (c) some of their special limitations and problems.

E. The need for, and value of, careful quantitative epidemiological studies of typhus in areas under consideration for control programs are stressed in order to select appropriate control measures and predict their effect on both immediate and long-range aspects of the problem.

F. Preliminary results of field studies in progress on the use of the living attenuated E strain vaccine in both epidemic and endemic typhus in Burundi and Bolivia are described. Practical and theoretical advantages of a typhus vaccine which imparts a durable immunity after a single dose are stressed, especially under conditions where effective louse control programs cannot be mounted and sustained. Both practical and theoretical problems of such a vaccine, i.e., reactions and stability of attenuation, are discussed.

ACKNOWLEDGEMENTS

The laboratory and field studies on the E strain typhus vaccine carried out by the Department of Microbiology of the University of Maryland, briefly and preliminarily reported here, were the results of the cumulative efforts of many dedicated people, both from the University and from collaborating organizations. When completed, these studies will be published in detail with appropriate individual and organizational acknowledgements. Various phases of these studies were carried out under the aegis of the Commission on Rickettsial Diseases of the Armed Forces Epidemiological Board, the Regional Office (AFRO) of the World Health Organization, the Pan American Health Organization and the Ministries of Health of Burundi and Bolivia and received partial financial support from contracts with the U.S. Army Research and Development Command, training grants from the National Institute of Allergy and Infectious Diseases, U.S. Public Health Service, the World Health Organization and the Pan American Health Organization.

REFERENCES

1. ZINSSER, H. Rats, Lice and History. Little, Brown and Co., Boston, 1934.
2. BIRAUD, Y. League of Nations Bull. *Health Org.* *10*:1, 1943.
3. NICOLLE, C., COMTE, C. & CONSEIL, E. *Compt. Rend. Acad. Sci.* *149*:486, 1909.
4. RICKETTS, H.T. & WILDER, R.M. *J. Am. Med. Assoc.* *54*:1373, 1910.
5. WOLBACH, S.B., TODD, J.L. & PALFREY, F.W. The Etiology and Pathology of Typhus. Harvard Univ. Press, Cambridge, 1922.
6. BRILL, N.E. *Am. J. Med. Sci.* *139*:484, 1910.
7. ZINSSER, H. *Am. J. Hyg.* *20*:513, 1934.
8. MOOSER, H. *Path. u. Bakt.* *16*:802, 1953.
9. MOSING, H. Office Internationale d'Hygiéne Public, Paris, *Bull. Mensuel* *30*:1715, 1938.
10. KOSTRZEWSKI, J. & WOJCIECHOWSKI, E. *Arch. Inst. Pasteur Tunis* *36*:379, 1959.
11. KOSTRZEWSKI, J. *Arch. Inst. Pasteur Tunis* *43*:357, 1966.
12. COMBIESCO, D., ZARNEA, G., BUZDUGAN, I. & IONESCO, H. *Arch. Inst. Pasteur Tunis* *36*:401, 1959.
13. ZDRODOVSKIJ, P.F. *Bull. World Health Org.* *31*:33, 1964.
14. GAON, J.A. & MURRAY, E.S. *Bull. World Health Org.* *35*:133, 1966.
15. MILOSOVIČOVÁ, A., TARABCÁK, M. WERNISCH, Z., KRATOCHVIL, I. & LUKÁCSOVÁ, V. *J. Hyg., Epidemiol., Microbiol. & Immunol.* *14*:393, 1970.
16. SNYDER, J.C. *Calif. Med.* *66*:3, 1947.
17. PHILIP, C.B. *Zentralbl. f. Bakt., Parasitenk., Infektionskr. u. Hyg.* *206*:343, 1968.
18. League of Nations. *Bull. Health Org. L. o. N.* *6*:205, 1937.
19. MONTOYA, J.A., JORDAN, M.E., KVAMME, L. QUIROS S., C., & FOX, J.P. *Am. J. Hyg.* *62*:255, 1955.
20. FREEMAN, G., CASTILLO SOLOGUREN, F. & ESPINOSA, H. *Am. J. Trop. Med.* *29*:71, 1949.
21. VIENTEMILLAS, F. Tratado sobre las Rickettsiasis y las Fiebres Exantematicas el Tifo Altiplanico. Escuela Tip. Salesiana, La Paz, Bolivia, 1944.
22. FREEMAN, G., VARELA, G., PLOTZ, H. & ORTIZ-MARIOTTE, C. *Am. J. Trop. Med.* *29*:63, 1949.
23. OLIVERA TORO, R. & ORTIZ-MARIOTTE, C. *Boletin Epidemiol. (Mexico)* *28*(1):5, 1964.
24. OLIVERA TORO, R. *Boletin Epidemiol. (Mexico)* *28*(1):11, 1964.
25. ORTIZ-MARIOTTE, C., MALO-JUVERA, F. & PAYNE, G.C. *Am. J. Pub. Health* *35*:1191, 1945.
26. ORTIZ-MARIOTTE, C. *Boletin Epidemiol. (Mexico)* *3*:9, 1945.
27. MARIÑO VELASQUEZ, F. & BERMEJO ORTEGA, R. *Revista Medica de Puno Vol. 1, No. 1,* Dec. 1954.

28. ORTIZ-MARIOTTE, C. *Pan Am. Sanitary Bur. Boletin 34*:236, 1953.
29. RISTORI, C., BOCCARDO, H., PINO, F., BORGOÑO, J. MANUEL & FRIZ, A. *Pan Am. Sanitary Bur. Boletin 43*:443, 1957.
30. ROJO, R. My Friend Che. (Translated by J. Casart). pp. 27-28, Dial Press, Inc., N.Y., 1968.
31. DAVIS, W.A., MALO JUVERA, F. & HERNANDEZ LIRA, P. *Am. J. Hyg. 39*:177, 1944.
32. SOPER, F.L., DAVIS, W.A., MARKHAM, F.S., RIEHL, L.A., & BUCK, P. *Arch. Inst. Pasteur Algerie 23*:183, 1945.
33. SOPER, F.L., DAVIS, W.A., MARKHAM, F.S. & RIEHL, L.A. *Am. J. Hyg. 45*:305, 1947.
34. DAVIS, W.A. *Am. J. Hyg. 46*:66, 1947.
35. World Health Organization. *World Health Org. Tech. Rep. Ser. No. 443*, 1970.
36. MILLER, R.N., WISSEMAN, C.L., JR., VERSCHUEREN, A. & FABRIKANT, I.B. (To be published.)
37. MURGATROYD, F. *Trans. Roy. Soc. Trop. Med. Hyg. 34*:1, 1940.
38. LONG, A.P. The Army Immunization Program. Ch. VIII in: Preventive Medicine in World War II. Vol. III. Personal Health Measures and Immunization, pp. 319-323. Medical Department, U.S. Army, 1955.
39. WISSEMAN, C.L., JR. PAHO/WHO First International Conf. on Vaccines against Viral and Rickettsial Dis. of Man. Pan Am. Health Org. Scientific Pub. No. 147, pp. 523-527, 1967.
40. WISSEMAN, C.L., JR. Proc. of the International Conf. on the Application of Vaccines against Viral, Rickettsial, and Bacterial Dis. of Man, 14-18 Dec. 1970. Pan Am. Health Org. Scientific Pub. No. 226, pp. 289-298, Wash., D.C. 1971.
41. WOODWARD, T.E., BLANC, G. & BALTAZARD, M. Unpublished data, personal communication.
42. DING, E. *Zeitschr. f. Hyg. u. Infektionskr. 124*:670, 1943.
43. ECKE, R.S., GILLIAM, A.G., SNYDER, J.C., YEOMANS, A., ZARAFONETIS, C.J. & MURRAY, E.S. *Am. J. Trop. Med. 25*:447, 1945.
44. SADUSK, J.F., JR. *J. Am. Med. Assoc. 133*:1192, 1947.
45. GILLIAM, A.G. *Am. J. Hyg. 44*:401, 1946.
46. DAVIS, W.A. *Ann. Int. Med. 34*:448, 1951.
47. LEVKOVICH. *Zh. Mikrobiol. Moscow I*:36, 1943.
48. WOHLRAB, R. & PATZER, G. *Münch. Med. Wchnschr. 91*(5/6):57, 1944.
49. TOPPING, N.H. *Am. J. Trop. Med. 24*:57, 1944.
50. MOOSER, H. *Schweiz. Med. Wchnschr. 76*:877, 1946.
51. SNYDER, J.C., MURRAY, E.S., YEOMANS, A., ZARAFONETIS, C.J.D. & WHEELER, C.M. *Am. J. Hyg. 49*:340, 1949.
52. CLAVERO, G. & PEREZ GALLARDO, F. *Rev. de Sanidad e Hig. Pub. 17*:1, 1943.
53. CLAVERO, G. & PEREZ GALLARDO, F. *Rev. de Sanidad e Hig. Pub. 18*:1, 1944.

54. FOX, J.P., EVERRITT, M.G. & ROBINSON, T.A. Atti del VI Cong. Internazionale di Microbiol. Roma, 6-12 Sept. 1953, Vol. 4, Section XI, pp. 51-65.
55. EVERRITT, M.G., BHATT, P.N. & FOX, J.P. *Am. J. Hyg.* *59*:60, 1954.
56. FOX, J.P., EVERRITT, M.G., ROBINSON, T.A. & CONWELL,D.P. *Am. J. Hyg.* *59*:74, 1954.
57. FOX, J.P. *Am. J. Publ. Health* *45*:1036, 1955.
58. FOX, J.P., MONTOYA, J.A., JORDAN, M.E. & ESPINOSA M. *Am. J. Hyg.* *61*:183, 1955.
59. FOX, J.P. *Am. J. Trop. Med. Hyg.* *5*:464, 1956.
60. FOX, J.P., JORDAN, M.E. & GELFAND, H.M. (Abstract) *Fed. Proc.* *16*:65, 1957.
61. FOX, J.P., JORDAN, M.E. & GELFAND, H.M. *J. Immunol.* *79*:348, 1957.
62. FOX, J.P. & JORDAN, M.E. *Bol. Oficina Sanitaria Panam.* *44*: 191, 1958.
63. MONTOYA, J.A., JORDAN, M.E., FOX, J.P. & GELFAND, H.M. *Proc. 6th Int. Congr. Trop. Med. & Malar.* *5*:612, 1959.
64. FOX, J.P., MONTOYA, J.A., JORDAN, M.E., CORREJO UBILLUS, J.R., GARCIA, J.L., ESTRADA, M.A. & GELFAND, H.M. *Arch. Inst. Pasteur Tunis* *36*:449, 1959.
65. ZDRODOWSKI, P. *Arch. Inst. Pasteur Tunis* *36*:501, 1959.
66. ZDRODOWSKI, P., GOLINEVITCH, H. HENIG, V., KEKTCHEEVA, N. & YABLONSKAYA, V. *Revue d'Immunolog., Paris* *30*:97, 1966.
67. ZDRODOWSKI, P. *Bull. Soc. Path. Exot.* *56*:822, 1963.
68. ZDRODOVSKII,P.F.*Probl. Virol.* *3*:141, 1958.
69. PSHENICHNOV, V.A., LEVASHOV, A.A., & NIKOLENKO, V. IA. *Probl. Virol.* *4*:64, 1959.
70. GOLINEVICH, E.M. & IABLONSKAIA, V.A. [Live exanthematous typhus vaccine from Strain E. of *R. prowazekii*]. In: Zdrodovskii, P.F. (ed): Voprosy Infektsionnoi Patologii i Immunologii, pp. 199-211, Medgiz, Moscow, 1963.
71. GOLINEVICH. E.M. & IABLONSKAIA, V. IA. [Immunization of people with live vaccine from Strain E of *Rickettsia prowazekii*]. In: Adrodovskii, P.F. (ed.): Voprosy Infektsionnoi Patologii i Immunologii, pp. 211-220, Medgiz, Moscow, 1963.
72. GOLINEVICH, E.M. & YABLONSKAYA, V.A. *J. Hyg., Epidemiol., Microbiol., & Immunol.* *7*:290, 1963.
73. URAKOV, N.N., PSHENICHNOV, V.A., SHCHETININ, V.P. & TERESHCHENKO, M.O. *Zh. Mikrobiol., Epidemiol. i Immunobiol.* *34*(7): 40, 1963.
74. IABLONSKAIA, V.A. *Vestn. Akad. Med. Nauk SSSR* *19*:61, 1964.
75. IABLONSKAIA, V.A. ET AL. *Vopr. Virusol.* *6*:680, 1965.
76. IMAM, I.Z.E., ALFY LABIB, EL RAI F. & HOSNY, A. *J. Egypt. Publ. Health Assoc.* *39*:33, 1964.
77. IMAM, I.Z.E., ALFY,LABIB,SHOUKRY,B., EL RAI, F. HEGAB, S. & HOSNY, A. *J. Egypt. Publ. Health Assoc.* *40*:483, 1965.

78. IMAM, I.Z.E., EL BATAWI, Y. AND ALFY,LABIB,*J. Egypt. Publ. Health Assoc.* *42:*47, 1967.
79. WISSEMAN, C.L., JR. ET AL. (To be published.)
80. WISSEMAN, C.L., JR., VERSCHUEREN, M., MILLER, R.N., FABRIKANT, I.B., & SWEENEY, G.W. (To be published.)
81. WISSEMAN, C.L., JR., VERSCHUEREN, A., MILLER, R.N., FABRIKANT, I.B. & SWEENEY, G.W. (To be published.)
82. PSHENICHNOV, V.A., LEVASHOV, A.A. & NIKOLENKO, V. IA. *Probl. of Virol.* *4:*64, 1959.
83. GENIG, V.A. *Probl. of Virol.* *4*(1):83, 1959.
84. WEISS, E. & DRESSLER, H.R. *J. Bact.* *75:*544, 1958.
85. FABRIKANT, IRENE B. The influence of prior irradiation on host susceptibility to infection with the attenuated E strain of *Rickettsia prowazekii*. Ph.D. Thesis, Univ. of Maryland, 1966.
86. PSHENICHNOV, V.A. *Probl. of Virol.* *6:*788, 1961.
87. GOLENIVICH, E.M. [Production, standardization, and control of live vaccine from Strain E, *Rickettsia prowazekii*]. In: Zdrodovskii, P.F. (ed.). Voprosy Infektsionnoi Patologii i Immunologii, pp. 187-195. Medgiz, Moscow, 1963.
88. SHKOLNIK, L. YA., & ZATULOVSKY, B.G. *Acta Virol.* *15:*102, 1971.
89. GAON, J. Attempts at virulence modification of "E" strain *R. prowazeki* by passage through body lice. Folia Medica Facultatis Medicinae Universitatis Saraeviensis, pp. 73-84, 1966.
90. BALAYEVA, N.W. *Vestnik Akademii Meditsinskikh Nauk SSSR* *24:* 51, 1969.
91. BALAYEVA, N.M. & NIKOLSKAYA, V.N. *Vestnik Akademii Meditsinskikh Nauk SSSR* *25:*17, 1970.
92. BALAYEVA, N.M. & NIKOLSKAYA. *Zh. Mikrobiol., Epidemiol. i Immunobiol.* *47:*36, 1970.
93. BALAYEVA, N.M. *J. Hyg. Epidemiol. Microbiol. Immunol.* *14:* 341, 1970.
94. PEREZ GALLARDO, F. & FOX, J.P. *Am. J. Hyg.* *48:*6, 1948.

THE POSSIBLE USE OF TEMPERATURE-SENSITIVE CONDITIONAL LETHAL MUTANTS FOR IMMUNIZATION IN VIRAL INFECTIONS

Frank Fenner

John Curtin School of Medical Research
Australian National University
Canberra, Australia

LIVE VIRUS VACCINES: HISTORICAL ASPECTS

South Africa and Australia were invaded and colonized by European man less than 200 years ago. In both places the settlers found ample grasslands and savannah-woodlands and an equable Mediterranean type of climate, and they soon introduced all the kinds of domestic animals that they had known in Europe. The impact of infectious diseases on these herds differed greatly in the two continents. Australia had been separated biogeographically from the rest of the world ever since the initial breakup of Pangaea, some 180 million years ago, and the only grazing animals there were marsupials, most of which were small in size and few in number. The rickettsial infection, Q fever, is the only disease that Australians have recognized as having been transferred to cattle and sheep from a marsupial reservoir host, and it caused trivial disease in the domestic as in the native animals. South Africa, on the other hand, is at the southern tip of a continent on which dwell a greater variety and a larger number of indigenous grazing animals than are found on any other continent. Wave after wave of novel infections, of differing virulence but often quite severe in the introduced species, emerged from this reservoir to assail one or another of the local domestic animals. In the 1930's, as virology began to emerge as a new science, the Ondersterpoort Veterinary Institute reacted to this challenge by developing a highly successful routine procedure for the production of new viral vaccines, which was applied to novel infectious agents even before they had been characterized. It consisted of adapting the novel virus or rickettsia to grow in chick embryos, in which it was subsequently passaged many times at an incubation temperature of 35°, for this had been found to promote the multiplication of most viruses in eggs (1). Periodical tests of its virulence were made in the stricken species of domestic animal, and it transpired that after 100 passages or so the virus was usually attenuated enough to allow it to be used as a live virus vaccine.

Live virus vaccines used in man have followed a similar line of development. Cowpox virus, doubtless contaminated with variola virus from time to time, was maintained by serial passage in the skins of cattle, with periodical transfers through human hosts; yellow fever virus was attenuated by serial passage in eggs and tissue culture; the same procedure was followed, with variations, for polioviruses, measles, rubella and mumps viruses. In essence, the empirical procedure was to pass the virus serially in a novel host or cultured cells, and usually at a reduced temperature of incubation -- sometimes, with "cold-adaptation", at a much reduced temperature. Periodic cautious tests for virulence, in primates or man, revealed progressive attenuation.

CONDITIONAL LETHAL MUTANTS

I would be the last to suggest that we should abandon an empirical and successful method for a "rational" approach that might not work. But it is worth considering if we can do better, more rapidly and certainly, if we decide that other live-virus vaccines are needed, either for human or for veterinary use. One possible "rational" procedure is deliberately to seek, and then stabilize, temperature-sensitive conditional lethal mutants as vaccine strains.

Geneticists have long recognized that in all organisms many mutations, both spontaneous and induced, were lethal, killing the organism at an early stage of development. The term *conditional lethal mutant* was introduced by Hadorn (2,3) to describe mutants of Drosophila that were either lethal, or allowed normal development to occur, depending upon growth conditions imposed by the experimenter. The conditions under which the mutation is lethal are called *restrictive*; conditions that allow development or multiplication to occur are called *permissive*. Conditional lethal mutants were introduced into phage research by Campbell (4) and greatly developed by Edgar and Epstein (5,6). Virtually all modern work on phage genetics makes extensive use of conditional lethal mutants.

The first deliberate and successful search for conditional lethal mutants of an animal virus was initiated in Canberra in 1960-61 by Dr. Mary McClain (7), who discovered that a proportion of the *u* mutants of rabbit pox virus (8) were host-dependent, in that they failed to replicate in PK cells, a continuous line derived from pig kidney. A little later, Cooper (9) recovered a group of temperature-sensitive mutants of poliovirus type 1. The trickle of papers published on conditional lethal mutants five years ago is now a veritable flood, almost all workers utilizing temperature-sensitive (*ts*) mutants, for animal cells equivalent to *sus* bacteria have yet to be recognized.

TEMPERATURE-SENSITIVE MUTANTS

What are temperature-sensitive mutants? In operational terms, they are conditional lethal mutants in which the condition that is manipulated is the temperature of incubation of the cells in which the virus is growing -- for one is concerned with temperature sensitivity of viral development rather than, necessarily, the sensitivity of viral infectivity to heat inactivation. At the molecular level, a temperature-sensitive mutation may involve no more than a change in a single nucleotide such that the corresponding polypeptide is altered in a way that allows it to function normally (or almost so) at the permissive temperature, but to be relatively or completely non-functional at the restrictive temperature.

As a class, temperature-sensitive mutants have several properties that should be noted: (a) Since temperature is a continuous variable, they rarely multiply as well as the wild type at the permissive temperature. (b) For the same reason, they may not be completely inactive at the restrictive temperature: the production of a few mutant progeny at the restrictive temperature is called "leak" or "leakiness." (c) Most single-step mutations revert to wild-type with a frequency of about 10^{-5}; if the mutation is temperature-sensitive, apparent "reversion" may occur with a higher frequency than this through certain mutations elsewhere in the same gene "correcting" the defect by a process called internal suppression. For vaccines one wants stable mutants; multiple mutants, or deletion mutants rather than mutants with base substitutions, may provide such stability.

The aspect of conditional lethal mutations that makes them valuable to the viral geneticist and physiologist is the fact that a single selective procedure, an elevated temperature of incubation or use of a restrictive host cell, can be used to select mutations in a very large number of different genes. Further, given a good plaque assay system, and especially with the help of some of the "mini-culture" systems and replica plating techniques now developed for animal virus culture, any virus will readily yield temperature-sensitive mutants. Temperature-sensitive mutants appeal to the virologist seeking to make vaccines because their defect, sensitivity of viral development to temperatures like that of the animal body, is likely to ensure that they are attenuated.

The Virulence of Temperature-Sensitive Mutants

Two characteristics relating to temperature are important. First, since they are selected for their failure to grow normally at body temperature, all temperature-sensitive mutants should in theory be attenuated. Second, it is possible to take advantage of the temperature gradients that exist in the animal body. For example, the skin temperature of man fluctuates around 33° and the temperature of the nasal cavity is 34°. Temperature-sensitive mutants can therefore be selected that grow well at such temperatures, but not at 37°. These facets of their behavior are so important in relation to vaccine production that I shall discuss them in some detail.

Experiments have been carried out with representatives of six genera of animal viruses, with the results set out in Table 1. All temperature-sensitive mutants tested, except one of the rabbit pox mutants and one of the rabies virus mutants, were less virulent than wild-type virus, usually much less virulent. In both these 'exceptions' the apparent virulence of the temperature-sensitive mutant may have been due to early reversion and subsequent dominance of wild-type virus; the rabbit pox virus case was not studied in detail and in the rabies virus example wild-type revertants were recovered from fatal cases. Three studies of the virulence of temperature-sensitive mutants, Semliki Forest virus, respiratory syncytial virus and influenza virus, will be described in greater detail.

Semliki Forest virus. Some years ago I carried out a number of experiments on the virulence of several temperature-sensitive mutants of Semliki Forest virus that were isolated and described by Tan *et al* (10). Doses as small as 10 PFU of wild-type virus were rapidly lethal after intracerebral inoculation into adult mice. In the experiments to be described, doses of 10^3 PFU of the mutants and 100 PFU of wild-type virus were inoculated into groups of nine mice that were subsequently held in animal rooms maintained at high (37°), moderate (15°) or low (4°) temperatures. The results are shown in Table 2. All mice infected with wild-type virus died in 3-5 days. None of the mice injected with temperature-sensitive mutants and held in a room at 37° were infected, for all survived and none were immune on challenge. At 15°, most mice inoculated with mutant strains survived, some with permanent paralysis of their hind limbs; at 4° there were several delayed deaths in mice inoculated with the two mutants (*ts* 9 and *ts* 10) having the highest cut-off temperature (37°), and occasional mice in some other mutant groups died. Clearly, all the mutants were much less virulent than the wild-type virus, and the survival of inoculated mice was related both to the cut-off temperature of the mutant and the temperature of the animal rooms (and thus the body temperature of the mice).

TABLE I

THE VIRULENCE OF TEMPERATURE-SENSITIVE MUTANTS

Virus	Temperature of Selection[a]	Tests in Animals				Ref.
		Species	Mutants	Number with Reduced Virulence	Active Immunity	
Rabbit pox	39.5°/34.5°	Rabbit Intradermal	7	6	+	10
Reovirus	37°/30°	Baby Hamster	6	6	. .	11
Rabies virus	40.5°/33°	Weanling Mice Intracerebral	2	1	+	12
Respiratory syncytial	39°/28°	Hamster Intranasal	4	4	+	13
Semliki Forest	38.3°/28°	Mouse Intracerebral	7	7	+	10
Influenza A (H_0N_1)	39°/33°	Mouse Intranasal	14	14	+	14
Influenza A (H_2N_2)	39°/32°	Hamster Intranasal	2	2	+	15
Influenza A (H_3N_2)	39°/32°	Hamster Intranasal	4	4	+	16

a - Temperature of selection = $\frac{\text{restrictive temperature}}{\text{permissive temperature}}$

TABLE II

THE RESPONSE OF MICE TO INTRACEREBRAL INJECTION WITH WILD-TYPE SEMLIKI FOREST VIRUS OR ITS *ts* MUTANTS

Virus	Cut-off Temperature[a]	Temperature of Animal Room		
		4°C	15°C	37°C
wild-type	39°	mst = 3.8 days[b]	mst = 4.5 days	mst = 4.1 days
ts 3	31°	(15)[c] 8 survivors	9 survivors	none infected
ts 5	34°	9 survivors	(10)(18) 6 survivors	none infected
ts 6	37°	9 survivors	9 survivors	none infected
ts 8	35°	(10)(10) 7 survivors	9 survivors	none infected
ts 9	37°	(4)(8)(8)(8)(9)(9)(10) 2 survivors	(21) 7 survivors	none infected
ts 10	37°	(7)(8)(10)(10)(10)(10) 2 survivors	(8) 8 survivors	none infected
ts 20	32°	(16) 7 survivors	9 survivors	none infected
rectal temperatures of mice		33°-36°	35.5°-37.5°	37°-39°

a - cut-off temperature = temperature at which the yield of virus was reduced by 99%.
b - mst = mean survival time (days).
c - values in brackets indicate day of death of an animal.

A more detailed study was made of the behavior of wild-type virus and the three more virulent mutants, *ts* 8, 9, 10 (Table 3). Mainly data obtained on the fourth day after infection are shown; assays made daily from the first until the eleventh day revealed the same pattern. In all cases, the titers were highest in mice maintained in the cold room, and at equivalent room temperatures the titers of the mutants in the brain were much lower than those of wild-type virus. Only the wild-type virus multiplied, and it to comparatively low titer, in mice maintained in the hot room; the mutants again failed to infect mice maintained at this temperature.

The serums of all mice were tested daily to determine when neutralizing antibody first appeared. There was some scatter, but in general some neutralizing antibody was found on the fourth or fifth day, although with *ts* 10, the mutant that multiplied least effectively of the viruses included in this experiment, neutralizing antibody appeared somewhat later. Interferon was detected in the brain on the second day in all groups except those infected with *ts* 10, when low levels were detected in one out of four mice tested, on the third day only. The experiments were not carried out in enough depth to allow for more than tentative conclusions, but compared with the body temperature of the mice and the temperature-sensitivity of viral development of the mutant involved, the host response was relatively unimportant in determining whether or not mice survived.

Respiratory syncytial virus. Several biological parameters were determined in hamsters inoculated intranasally with wild-type respiratory syncytial virus and each of four temperature-sensitive mutants (13). All the mutants multiplied to lower titers than wild-type in turbinates and lungs; no virus was recovered from hamsters inoculated with *ts* 4 but some multiplication must have occurred since there was a serologic response and active immunization. The two leaky mutants, *ts* 2 and *ts* 3, grew to some extent in the lungs; the other two were not detected there, and all four mutants were genetically stable *in vitro* and *in vivo*.

Influenza virus. Mackenzie (14) found that each of fourteen temperature-sensitive mutants of influenza strain WSN [A(H_0N_1)] was less virulent than was wild-type virus after intranasal inoculation. Analyzing this data, Mills *et al.*, (18) showed that there was a significant correlation between virulence and the cut-off temperature of the mutants.

TABLE III

SOME FEATURES OF INFECTION IN MICE INOCULATED INTRACEREBRALLY WITH WILD-TYPE SEMLIKI FOREST VIRUS OR ITS *ts* MUTANTS

Virus	Temperature of Animal Room	Mortality	Viral Content of Brain on Day 4 (log PFU/Brain)[a]	Serum Neutralizing Antibody First Detected (Day)[a]	Interferon Present in Brain on Day 2
Wild-type	4°	mst. 3.8 days	7.5; 7.7	-	+
	15°	mst. 4.0 days	7.0; 7.5	-,4	+
	37°	mst. 4.5 days	5.2; 6.2	-,4	±
ts 8	4°	(7)[b](11)(14);6 survivors	3.6; 3.8	4,5	+
	15°	9 survivors	3.6; 1.6	5,5	±
	37°	none infected	0 ; 0	-	-
ts 9	4°	(7)(7)(8)(8)(9)(11); 3 survivors	4.3; 6.6	5,5	±
	15°	(9)(11)(12)(14)(14); 4 survivors	3.1; 4.8	4,4	+
	37°	none infected	0 ; 0	-	-
ts 10	4°	(7)(8)(12); 6 survivors	3.2; 2.5	7,8	-
	15°	(13); 8 survivors	2.2; 2.4	4,7	-
	37°	none infected	0 ; 0	-	-

a - Values for two mice sampled for virus and interferon in brain and antibody in serum.

b - Values in brackets indicate day of death of an animal.

mst = mean survival time.

TABLE IV

IN VITRO AND *IN VIVO* PROPERTIES OF *ts* MUTANTS OF RESPIRATORY SYNCYTIAL VIRUS
(From Reference 13)

Virus	HeLa Cells				Hamsters			
	Suppression of Plaques at			Leakiness	Viral Growth in		Serologic Response	Active Immunity
	37°	38°	39°		Turbinates	Lungs		
Wild-type	0	0	0		+++	+++	+++	+++
ts 1	++	+++		0	++	0	++	+++
ts 2	+++	+++		++	+	+	++	+++
ts 3	++	+++		+	++	++	++	+++
ts 4	+++	+++		0	0	0	++	+++

Searching for strains to make a live vaccine, Mills and Chanock (15) inoculated two stable mutants of influenza A2 [A (H_2N_2)] into hamsters. *Ts* 1 grew very poorly in their lungs and *ts* 2 somewhat better, but still less than wild-type virus. A few revertants were found in the lungs of hamsters injected with *ts* 2, but the proportion did not increase during the course of the disease and seldom exceeded 1 percent. Infection of mice with the mutants produced substantial protection against challenge with wild-type virus. Subsequently, Chanock (16) carried out mixed infection experiments with *ts* 1 and *ts* 2 [A (H_2N_2)] and wild-type Hong Kong virus [A (H_3N_2)] and recovered four *ts* recombinants with the Hong Kong hemagglutinin (H_3); three from *ts* 1 and one from *ts* 2. Unexpectedly, each of the four recombinants had a different pattern of temperature restriction and in pairwise combinations they fell into four complementation groups. Assuming that recombination had occurred by reassortment of pieces of the fragmented genome of influenza virus, these results suggest that the original $A(H_2N_2)$ mutant *ts* 1 had temperature-sensitive lesions in three different genes. All of the recombinants were of decreased virulence in hamsters; as in Mackenzie's experiments, there was a correlation between cut-off temperature and virulence. In eggs and cultured cells the temperature-sensitive recombinants were stable; revertants were recovered from the hamster lungs, but never constituted more than a minority of the yield.

Human Vaccination with Temperature-Sensitive Mutants

The only vaccination trials carried out with temperature-sensitive mutants are limited experiments with respiratory syncytial virus and influenza virus.

<u>Respiratory syncytial virus</u>. This ubiquitous monotypic virus can produce severe bronchiolitis in very young infants, and trivial or inapparent reinfections thereafter. All adults have serum antibody, which is probably not related to protection. Twenty-one men with low levels of nasal secretory antibody were selected out of 100 volunteers (19). Nine were challenged by intranasal inoculation of mutant *ts* 1. Only three shed virus, for a few days only and to a very low titer, whereas six of eight men inoculated with wild-type respiratory syncytial virus shed virus, to a higher titer and over a more prolonged period. None of the men challenged with *ts* 1 was sick; five of the eight men inoculated with wild-type virus had an upper respiratory illness. There was a measurable immunologic response in only one out of the nine volunteers inoculated with *ts* 1 but seven of them subsequently challenged with wild-type respiratory syncytial virus were protected, virologically and clinically.

Influenza virus. Several of the *ts* recombinants and wild-type Hong Kong virus were tested by intranasal inoculation of seronegative volunteers (16). Some selected results are illustrated in Table 5. The recombinant *ts* 1-A, which had failed to multiply in the hamster lung, was also clearly too 'attenuated' (probably too temperature-sensitive) to infect adult human volunteers. Recombinant *ts* 1-E, on the other hand, appeared to meet most of the criteria required for a satisfactory vaccine strain. It produced infection without illness, both serum and nasal antibody responses were satisfactory, and there was complete protection against re-infection five weeks later.

DISCUSSION

In a sense, the 'rational' approach to the selection of viral vaccines for human use has come too late. Accumulated experience is rightly a factor of great importance in the minds of licensing authorities, and live virus vaccines have already been produced by empirical methods and used on a large scale for most of the common generalized human viral diseases; smallpox, yellow fever, poliomyelitis, measles, rubella and mumps. Apart from still wholly hypothetical requirements such as live virus vaccines against hepatitis or cancer, and possible needs for particular groups or localities, e.g., military personnel or local arbovirus diseases, the future demand in the field of human medicine centers upon protection against respiratory viruses. The demands for safety and efficiency of new vaccines will undoubtedly be higher in the future than they have been in the past, partly because the diseases are less threatening and partly because of virological sophistication. In addition, vaccines against respiratory infections present special problems which include the following: (a) Even after natural infections, immunity to re-infection is relatively transient, rather than virtually lifelong as in the generalized infections, so that repeated vaccination may be necessary. (b) With respiratory syncytial virus, the age-group at serious risk comprises very young infants, a particularly difficult group to test. (c) With influenza, quite the most serious respiratory disease, the antigenic pattern of the viruses is constantly undergoing minor changes by antigenic drift and we can anticipate that at intervals of a decade or so major antigenic shifts will continue to occur in the future as they have done during the last half century. Vaccines will therefore have to continually updated, i.e., changed in the nature of the envelope antigens they contain.

Public health authorities are faced with substantial problems in deciding upon future policy as to the extent to which vaccination against respiratory viral infections is justifiable. There would seem to be no doubt that it is essential to be prepared for

TABLE V

CHALLENGE EXPERIMENTS IN SERONEGATIVE HUMAN VOLUNTEERS WITH WILD-TYPE HONG KONG [A(H_3N_2)] INFLUENZA VIRUS AND TEMPERATURE-SENSITIVE RECOMBINANTS [A(H_3N_2)] (From Reference 16)

Virus	Cut-off Temperature	Response in Volunteers					Challenge [A(H_3N_2)]wild-type		
		Infected/Tested	Illness		Antibody Rise		Virus Shed/Tested	Illness	
			Any	Influenzal	Serum	Nasal		Any	Influenzal
ts 1-A	37°	0/13	0	0	0	0			
ts 1-E	38°	16/17	5	0	x10[a]	x8	0/12	0	0
wild-type	>40°	19/21	14	11	x32	x12	18/21	14	11

a - x10 = tenfold increase in antibody titer.

future pandemic influenza. Inactivated vaccines have been disappointing and there are theoretical reasons for preferring intranasal inoculation to parenteral, probably with live virus vaccines because of considerations of dosage and speed of preparation of new vaccines in emergency situations. Our present effort should therefore be aimed at getting a basic strain that has the following desirable qualities: failure to produce disease but capacity to infect and produce antibody in susceptible individuals; genetic stability in its virulence; and the capacity to grow to high titer in a cell system acceptable to licensing authorities. I do not believe that we can anticipate the antigenic make up of the next pandemic strain, but with this basic strain the requisite reassortment virus could be rapidly produced.

For other respiratory viral infections the case for general vaccination is less convincing. Respiratory syncytial virus is a serious disease in the very young, but the relatively trivial symptoms of the common cold and the multiplicity to serotypes of agents like rhinoviruses, coronaviruses, etc., hardly justify the production of vaccines. Vaccines will continue to be needed for specially vulnerable groups (e.g., military personnel) and the approach I have described provides a rational way of producing them.

ACKNOWLEDGEMENT

This paper was prepared while the author was a Fogarty Scholar-in-Residence, Fogarty International Center, N.I.H.

REFERENCES

1. BEVERIDGE, W.I.B. & BURNET, F.M. *Med. Res. Council Spec. Rept. Sci.* *256*, 1946.
2. HADORN, E. *Adv. Genet.* *4*:53, 1951.
3. HADORN, E. "Developmental Genetics and Lethal Factors", p. 118, Methuen, London, 1961.
4. CAMPBELL, A. *Virology* *14*:22, 1961.
5. EPSTEIN, R.H., BOLLE, A., STEINBERG, C.M., KELLENBERGER, E. ET AL. *Cold Spring Harbor Symp. Quant. Biol.* *28*:375, 1963.
6. EDGAR, R.S. Conditional lethals, in: "Phage and the Origins of Molecular Biology", p. 166. (Eds. J. Cairns, G.S. Stent and J.D. Watson), Cold Spring Harbor Lab. N.Y., 1966.
7. McCLAIN, M.E. *Aust. J. Exp. Biol. Med. Sci.* *43*:31, 1965.
8. GEMMELL, A. AND FENNER, F. *Virology* *11*:219, 1960.
9. COOPER, P.D. *Virology* *22*:186, 1964.
10. FENNER, F. Unpublished data, 1965.

11. IKEGAMI, N. & GOMATOS, P.J. *Virology* *36*:447, 1968.
12. CLARK, H.F. & KOPROWSKI, H. *J. Virol.* *7*:295, 1971.
13. WRIGHT, P.F., WOODEND, W.G. & CHANOCK, R.M. *J. Inf. Dis.* *122*:501, 1970.
14. MACKENZIE, J.S. *Brit. Med. J.* *2*:757, 1969.
15. MILLS, J. & CHANOCK, R.M. *J. Inf. Dis.* *123*:145, 1971.
16. CHANOCK. R.M. Unpublished data, 1972.
17. TAN, K.B., SAMBROOK, J.F. & BELLETT, A.J.D. *Virology* *38*:427, 1969.
18. MILLS, J., CHANOCK, R.M., ALLING, D.W. *Brit. Med. J.* *4*:690, 1969.
19. WRIGHT, P.F., MILLS, J. & CHANOCK, R.M. *J. Inf. Dis.* *124*:505, 1971.

GENETIC CONTROL AND IMMUNITY

Edna Mozes, G.M. Shearer and Michael Sela

Department of Chemical Immunology
The Weizmann Institute of Science
Rehovoth, Israel

For more than half a century a correlation has been known to exist between the ability to respond to an antigen and the genetic constitution of an individual. In 1916, Cooke and van der Veer provided experimental evidence that inheritance plays a role in some forms of human sensitization, e.g., hay fever, bronchial asthma, gastro-enteritis and urticaria (1). Furthermore, these investigators concluded that this phenomenon is inherited as a dominant characteristic, involving the ability of an individual to form specific antibodies, and is not due to transmission of sensitization from parent to offspring. Thus, the ability of an individual to elicit an immune response to a given immunogen is genetically affected, although the immune state of that individual is not itself an inherited characteristic. Recent analyses of animal and human disease states suggest that genes which control immune responsiveness affect susceptibility or resistance to certain diseases (2). In order to understand these phenomena in humans, experimental models using inbred mice (in which the genetic parameters can be controlled) and synthetic polypeptide antigens (in which the chemical structure can be defined) have been studied.

Evidence for determinant-specific genetic control of antibody response in inbred strains of mice has been obtained with synthetic multichain polypeptide antigens, in which short peptides containing glutamic acid and tyrosine, histidine, or phenylalanine were attached to the amino acid termini of multichain poly-DL-alanine (3,4). For example, C57 black mice are good producers of antibodies against the tyrosine-containing polymer while responding poorly to the histidine-containing polymer; the situation is completely reversed in CBA mice. In short, the genetic factors can discriminate between tyrosine, histidine, and phenylalanine in the determinant. These genetic differences are dominant, unigenic, quantitative, and determinant-specific. The ability of mice to respond to the above antigens is a genetic trait closely linked to the major (H-2) histocompatibility locus in the IXth linkage group.

Genetic control of immunological responsiveness has also been demonstrated for a series of branched chain synthetic polypeptides built on multichain poly-L-proline, (Pro--L) (5,6). The immune response of inbred mice to the "Pro--L" series of immunogens differs from the response of the same mouse strains to the polypeptides built on poly-DL-alanine, even though the same short sequences of tyrosine or phenylalanine and glutamic acid were attached to the polypeptide side chains in both series. Genetic analysis of the immune response to poly-L-(Tyr,Glu)-poly-L-Pro--poly-LLys, (T,G)-Pro--L, in SJL (high responder) and DBA/1 (low responder) mice as well as in the F1 and backcross recombinants, indicated that the ability to respond to this synthetic immunogen is not linked to H-2 (6).

Different inbred strains of mice may produce similar amounts of antibodies against the same protein, but these antibodies could be specific for different determinants within the complex immunogen. Studies of the genetic control of immune response to poly-L-(Phe,G)-poly-L-Pro--poly-L-Lys, (Phe,G)-Pro--L (Fig. 1) have verified this hypothesis. DBA/1 mice, which are high responders to (Phe,G)-A--L, produce antibodies to the (Phe,G) part of the polypeptide, whereas SJL mice make antibodies to the Pro--L region of the same immunogen (Table 1). There is no linkage between the ability to respond to the Pro--L portion of (Phe,G)-Pro--L and H-2, whereas the response potential for the (Phe,G) part of the same immunogen is closely linked to the H-2 region (6). These results indicate that two distinct gene loci regulate the ability to respond to (Phe,G)-Pro--L.

Direct evidence for genetic control at the level of unique antigenic determinants of native proteins came from a recent study on the "loop" peptide of lysozyme. Although most inbred mice responded well to hen egg white lysozyme, strains were found which did not respond to the "loop" region (residues 60-83) of this protein (7). As shown in Table 2, SJL mice are low responders to the "loop" peptide when it is attached to A--L,Pro--L or when it is within lysozyme. In contrast, the DBA/1 strain responds well to "loop", irrespective of the macromolecule to which it is attached. The genetic control of immune response to "loop" is similar to the control of responsiveness to (Phe,G). Thus SJL mice are low responders to "loop"-A--L as they are to (Phe,G)-A--L. However, they are high responders to "loop"-Pro--L as well as to (Phe,G)-Pro--L, but the antibodies produced are specific for Pro--L. Althouth SJL mice do respond to lysozyme, the response is specific

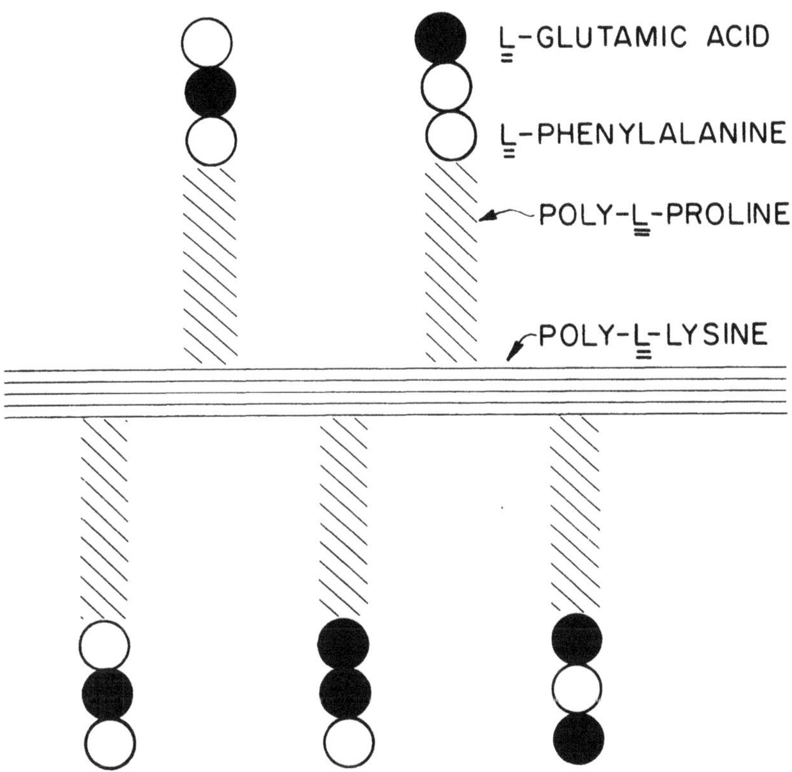

Fig. 1 Schematic diagram of a multichain copolymer composed of a backbone of poly-L-lysine to which are attached sidechains of poly-L-proline, elongated with peptides of L-tyrosine and L-glutamic acid. This polymer is denoted multi-copoly(Phe,Glu)-polyPro--polyLys, and abbreviated as (Phe,G)-Pro--L.

TABLE I

IMMUNE RESPONSES OF INTACT SJL AND DBA/1 MICE TO MULTICHAIN SYNTHETIC POLYPEPTIDES

Immunogen	Titering Antigen	
	(T,G)-Pro--L	(Phe,G)-A--L
	SJL Strain	
(Phe,G)-Pro--L	High	Low
(T,G)-Pro--L	High	-
(Phe,G)-A--L	-	Low
	DBA/1 Strain	
(Phe,G)-Pro--L	Low	High
(T,G)-Pro--L	Low	-
(Phe,G)-A--L	-	High

TABLE II

IMMUNE RESPONSES OF INTACT SJL AND DBA/1 MICE TO THE "LOOP" PEPTIDE OF LYSOZYME

Immunized with:	Lysozyme		"Loop"-A--L		"Loop"-Pro--L	
Assayed with:	Lysozyme	"Loop"	Lysozyme	(T,G)-A--L	Lysozyme	(T,G)-Pro--L
SJL Strain	High	Low	Low	Low	Low	High
DAB/1 Strain	High	High	High	Low	High	Low

for determinants other than "loop" which have not been defined.

In order to better understand the mechanism(s) by which genetic regulation of responsiveness operates, it is important to establish which functional populations of immunocompetent cells exhibit the defect. To do this, it is first necessary to determine how the defect is expressed by the cells themselves. Since the genetic defect is quantitative, i.e., the low responders do generate reduced but detectable responses, expression of the defect could be reflected in a lower number of antigen-sensitive units stimulated by the immunogen. The objective of the studies summarized here was to determine whether the low immune responses to the (Phe,G) and Pro--L immunopotent regions of (Phe,G)-Pro--L and (Phe,G)-A--L in SJL and DBA/1 mice could be correlated with a reduced number of detectable splenic antigen-sensitive units in the respective low responder strain; and if so, to establish whether such a reduction in frequency could be attributed to a thymus- or marrow-derived population of cells. An antigen-sensitive unit is defined as the minimal functional cellular unit necessary for generating an immune response (8). For thymus-dependent immunogens, such an immunocompetent unit of response is made up of at least a bone marrow-derived precursor of antibody-forming cells and a thymus-derived cell considered to play some helper role in the immune system (9-11). The frequencies of antigen-sensitive units relevant to these synthetic immunogens have been estimated in mouse spleens and in mixtures of thymocytes and marrow cells by limiting dilution assays (12-15). This analysis is based on the fact that a critically low number of transplanted cells will not generate a donor-derived immune response in lethally irradiated recipients, since the least frequent precursor cell type relevant for the response is not contained in the inoculum. Conversely, a relatively high number of cells injected will contain <u>all</u> required precursor types, and a donor-derived response will result. By plotting the percentage of positive responses in recipients as a function of the number of cells transferred, a curve is obtained which conforms to the predictions of the Poisson model. Therefore, this statistical approach has been used to describe the theoretical probability that antigen-sensitive units contained in a given number of spleen cells generate an immune response.

SJL and DBA/1 mice were exposed to 700-800 R of X-irradiation and injected with graded numbers (1×10^6 - 4×10^7) of spleen cells from non-immunized or immunized syngeneic donors. Recipients were immunized intraperitoneally with 10 μg (Phe,G)-Pro--L, (T,G)-Pro--L or (Phe,G)-A--L in complete Freund's adjuvant 24 hours later. Sera of individual recipients were collected two weeks after cell transfer (at the time of peak antibody titers), and assayed for (Phe,G)- and Pro--L-specific antibodies by passive microhemagglutination, using sheep erythrocytes coated with

(Phe,G)-A--L or with (T,G)-Pro--L (13). Sera from control animals either exhibited no detectable titers or gave responses detectable at a dilution not greater than 1:4. Sera were considered to be positive or negative, depending on whether or not antibodies specific for (Phe,G) and/or Pro--L were detected at a dilution greater than 1:4. Results of these limiting dilution experiments are summarized graphically in Figs. 2 and 3. The observed frequencies are indicated by the points, and the curves give the expected frequency patterns, assuming a single-hit Poisson model. The limiting frequencies of antigen-sensitive precursor cells calculated from all the data (i.e., the cell inoculum necessary to generate a response in 63 percent of the recipients) are also shown in the figures. In all experiments, as the spleen cell inoculum was increased, a corresponding increase was observed in the fraction of positive recipient sera titered with (Phe,G)-A--L and (T,G)-Pro--L, in both mouse strains. When (Phe,G)-Pro--L was used as the immunogen with spleen cells from non-immunized SJL donors (see upper part of Fig. 2), a six-fold difference was detected in frequencies of splenic precursors for the (Phe,G) and Pro--L specificities (13). A greater frequency of precursors was detected for the Pro--L than for the (Phe,G) determinant. For spleen cells from SJL donors preimmunized with (Phe,G)-Pro--L (see lower part of Fig. 2), the relative number of detected precursors specific for (Phe,G) was 15 times less than that for Pro--L when these determinants are carried on the same immunogenic macromolecule (13). In contrast, the difference between the frequencies of (Phe,G)- and Pro--L-specific precursors in the spleens of non-immunized and immunized DBA/1 donors were respectively 4.5 and 5.5 (see Fig. 3). In this case, the frequency of responses specific for (Phe,G) (to which DBA/1 are high responders) was consistently higher than that obtained for Pro--L (13). These results indicate that the genetic control of immunity to the synthetic polypeptide antigen investigated is directly correlated with the relative number of precursor cells reactive with the immunogen in high and low responder strains. Similar results were obtained using (T,G)-Pro--L and (Phe,G)-A--L as the immunogens (12,15). For these immunogens, the (Phe,G) and Pro--L immunopotent regions are carried on separate molecules. A higher response frequency was observed in the high responder SJL than in the low responder DBA/1 strain for (T,G)-Pro--L. Conversely, for (Phe,G)-A--L, a greater frequency of precursors was detected in the spleens of DBA/1 (high responder to this immunogen) than in those of SJL (low responder) donors (data not shown).

Since expression of the genetic control of immune response has been demonstrated at the cellular level, it is important to establish which functional populations of immunocompetent cells exhibit the defect. In order to establish whether thymus and/or marrow cells play a role in expression of the genetic control of immune responses to the three immunogens, it was necessary to demonstrate that cell-to-cell interaction is required for (Phe,G) and Pro--L

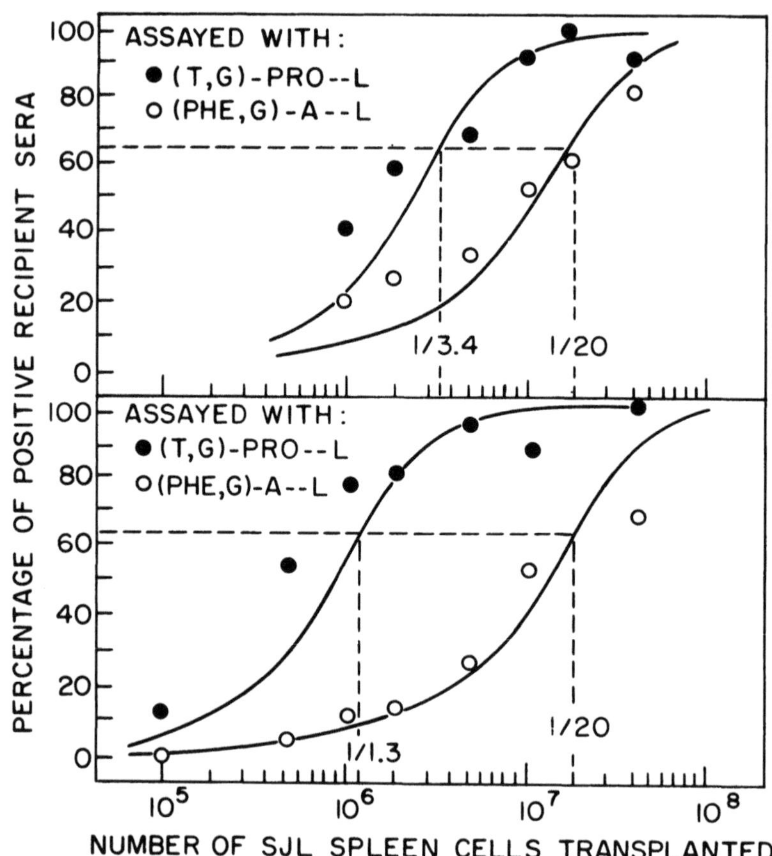

Fig. 2 Percentage of positive sera in SJL recipients when assayed with (Phe,G)-A--L (o) or (T,G)-Pro--L (●) after irradiation and injection of (Phe,G)-Pro--L and graded numbers of spleen cells from non-immunized (upper) or immunized (lower) syngeneic donors.

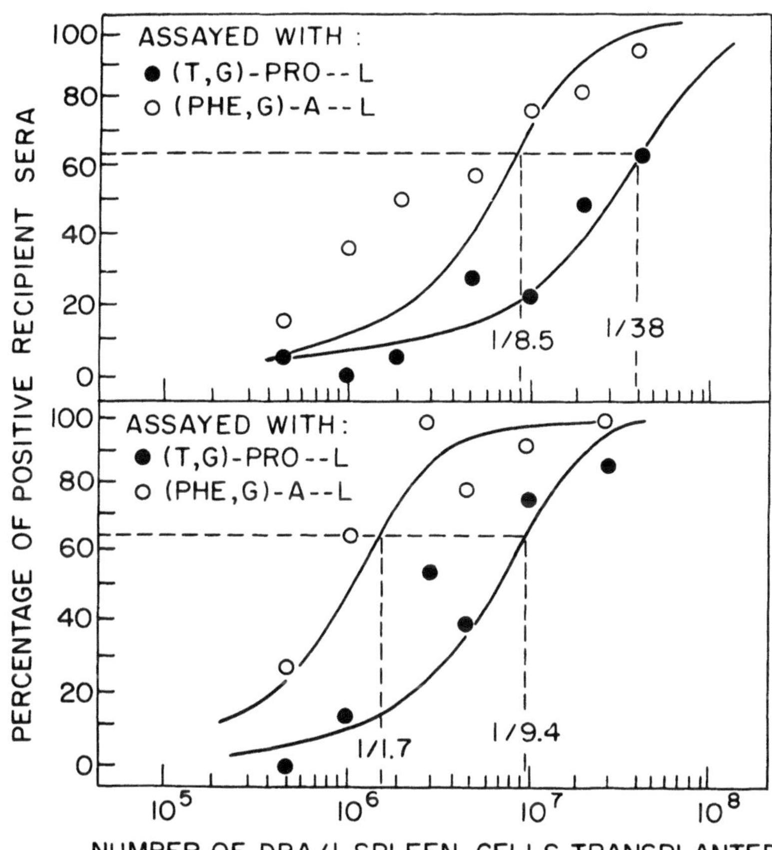

Fig. 3 Percentage of positive sera in DBA/1 recipients when assayed with (Phe,G)-A--L (o) or (T,G)-Pro--L (•) after irradiation and injection of (Phe,G)-Pro--L and graded numbers of spleen cells from non-immunized (upper) or immunized (lower) syngeneic donors.

responses. Irradiated SJL and DBA/1 mice were injected with thymocytes, or bone marrow cells, or with a mixture containing thymus and marrow cells taken from syngeneic donors, and immunized with (Phe,G)-Pro--L, (T,G)-Pro--L or (Phe,G)-A--L 24 hours later. Two weeks after cell transfer, the recipients were bled and their sera individually assayed for (Phe,G)- and Pro--L-specific antibodies. As shown in Table 3, thymocytes or marrow cells alone did not generate detectable immune responses to any of the three immunogens. In contrast, an inoculum containing a mixture of these cell types generated (Phe,G)- and Pro--L-specific responses in most of the recipients. Therefore, thymus-marrow cooperation appears to be necessary for generating antibody responses in recipient mice immunized with these three immunogens in complete Freund's adjuvant (14,15).

In order to determine whether these genetic defects are reflected in the thymus- or marrow-derived populations of immunocompetent cells, dilution transfer experiments were performed in which a constant and excess number of one cell type was mixed with graded and limiting numbers of the complementary cell type. Irradiated SJL and DBA/1 mice were injected with graded inocula of syngeneic marrow cells (5×10^4 - 2×10^7) to which an excess of 10^8 syngeneic thymocytes had been added. The recipients were immunized with (Phe,G)-Pro--L and their sera assayed as described above. These limiting dilution data are shown in the upper portions of Figs. 4 and 5. Differences of about five-fold were observed in the frequencies of (Phe,G) and Pro--L responses in both mouse strains, similar to the results obtained with limiting inocula of spleen cells from non-immunized donors (14). For the SJL strain, which is the low responder to (Phe,G), five times as many relevant marrow precursors were detected for the Pro--L as for the (Phe,G) specificity. The calculated frequencies were $1/1.7 \times 10^6$ and $1/7.3 \times 10^6$, respectively. For the DBA/1 strain (low responder to Pro--L), one precursor was detected in 1.9×10^6 marrow cells for (Phe,G), whereas an average of 6.5×10^6 marrow cells had to be injected in order to detect one Pro--L marrow precursor (14). Thus, the marrow cell limiting dilution data indicate that the low response of the SJL strain to (Phe,G) and of DBA/1 mice to Pro--L can be accounted for by a five-fold reduced number of monospecific precursors detected in the bone marrow of these two mouse strains.

In order to estimate the relative numbers of thymus cells stimulated by (Phe,G)-Pro--L, graded inocula of syngeneic thymocytes (0.5-100×10^6) were mixed with 2×10^7 syngeneic bone marrow cells, and injected into groups of irradiated SJL and DBA/1 mice. The recipients were immunized with (Phe,G)-Pro--L, and their sera individually assayed for (Phe,G) and Pro--L responses, as described above. The results are summarized in the lower parts of Figs. 6 and 7. In contrast to the results obtained with limiting inocula

TABLE III

INTERACTION BETWEEN THYMOCYTES AND BONE MARROW CELLS IN IMMUNE RESPONSES TO MULTICHAIN SYNTHETIC POLYPEPTIDES IN SJL AND DBA/1 MICE

Immunogen	Mouse Strain	Thymocytes Injected	Marrow Cells Injected	Percentage of Positive Sera in Recipients Assayed With:	
				(T,G)-Pro--L	(Phe,G)-A--L
(Phe,G)-Pro--L	SJL	-	-	-	-
		0	2×10^7	6	0
		1×10^8	2×10^7	100	95
(Phe,G)-Pro--L	DBA/1	1×10^8	0	0	0
		0	2×10^7	6	11
		1×10^8	2×10^7	86	91
(T,G)-Pro--L	SJL	7.5×10^7	0	0	-
		0	1.5×10^7	8	-
		7.5×10^7	1.5×10^7	100	-
(T,G)-Pro--L	DBA/1	7.5×10^7	0	0	-
		0	1.5×10^7	18	-
		7.5×10^7	1.5×10^7	73	-
(Phe,G)-A--L	SJL	1×10^8	0	-	16
		0	2×10^7	-	19
		1×10^3	2×10^7	-	82
(Phe,G)-A--L	DBA/1	1×10^8	0	-	0
		0	2×10^7	-	17
		1×10^8	2×10^7	-	100

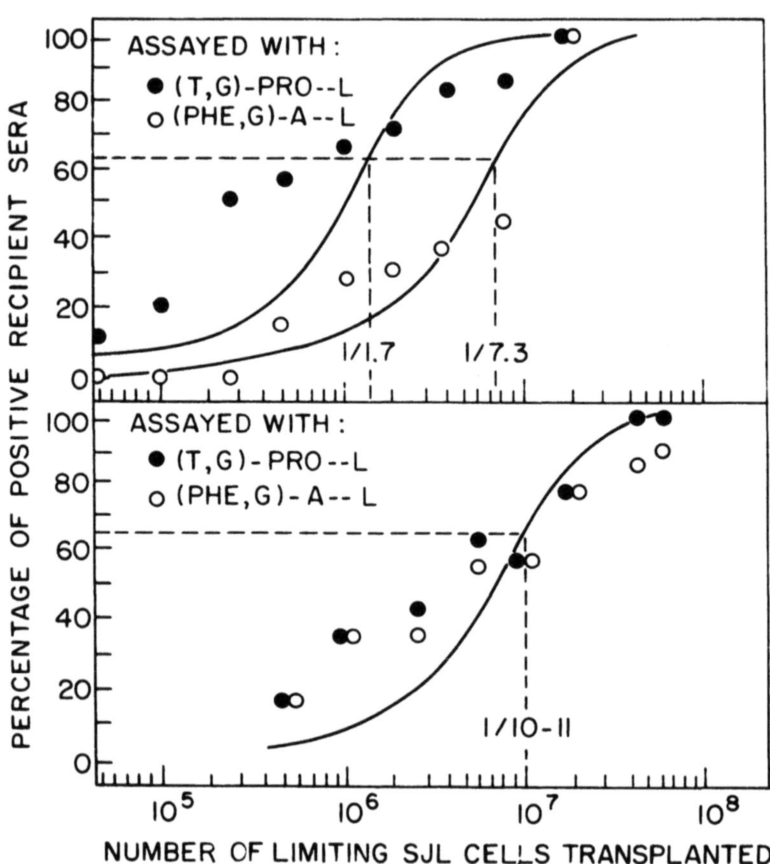

Fig. 4 Percentage of positive sera in SJL recipients when assayed with (Phe,G)-A--L (o) or (T,G)-Pro--L (•) after irradiation and injection of (Phe,G)-Pro--L either with 10^8 thymocytes and graded numbers of bone marrow cells (upper), or with 2 x 10^7 bone marrow cells and graded numbers of thymocytes (lower) from syngeneic non-immunized donors.

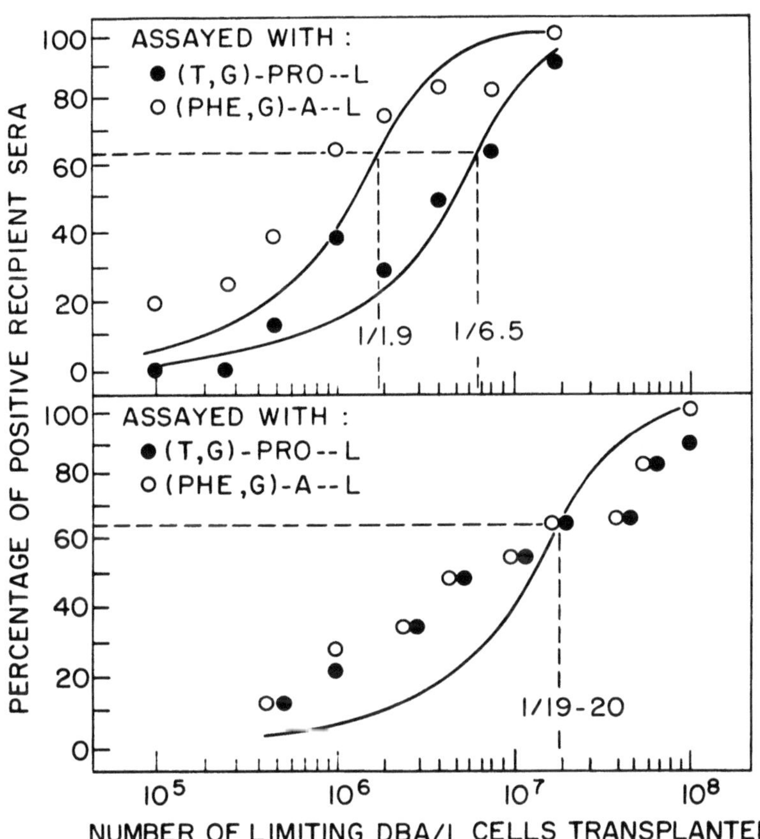

Fig. 5 Percentage of positive sera in DBA/1 recipients when assayed with (Phe,G)-A--L (o) or (T,G)-Pro--L (•) after irradiation and injection of (Phe,G)-Pro--L either with 10^8 thymocytes and graded numbers of bone marrow cells (upper), or with 2 x 10^7 bone marrow cells and graded numbers of thymocytes (lower) from syngeneic non-immunized donors.

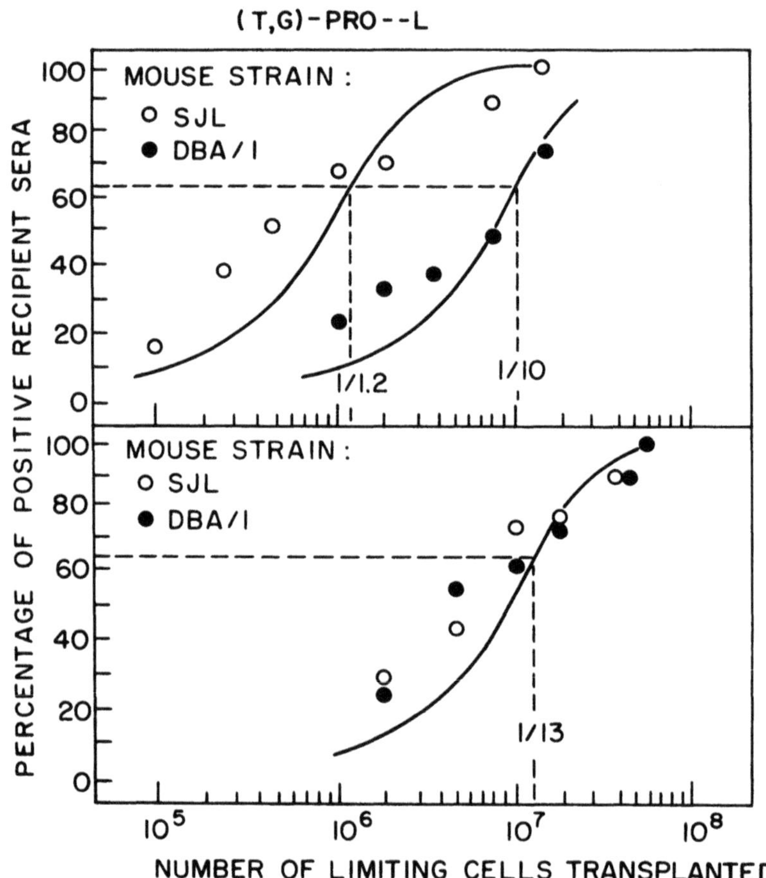

Fig. 6 Percentage of positive sera in SJL (o) or DBA/1 (●) recipients when assayed with (T,G)-Pro--L after irradiation and injection of (T,G)-Pro--L either with 10^8 thymocytes and graded numbers of bone marrow cells (upper) or with 2 x 10^7 bone marrow cells and graded numbers of thymocytes (lower) from syngeneic non-immunized donors.

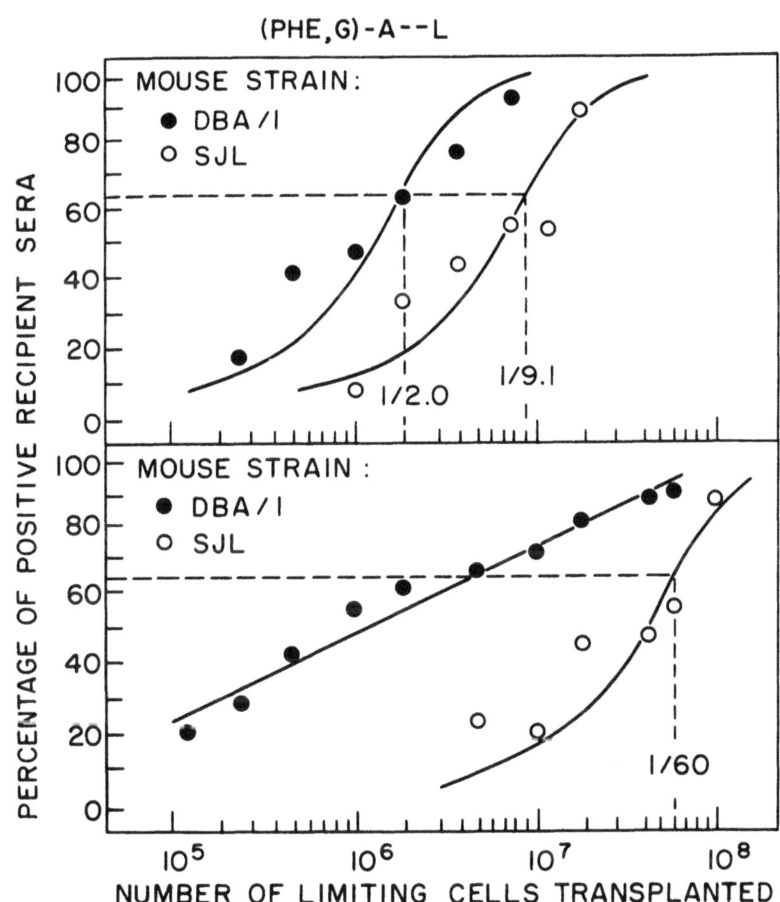

Fig. 7 Percentage of positive sera in SJL (o) or DBA/1 (•) recipients when assayed with (Phe,G)-A--L after irradiation and injection of (Phe,G)-A--L either with 10^8 thymocytes and graded numbers of bone marrow cells (upper) or with 2 x 10^7 bone marrow cells and graded numbers of thymocytes (lower) from syngeneic non-immunized donors.

of spleen or marrow cells, no significant differences were detected when the responses were limited by the number of thymocytes transferred for either specificity in these two mouse strains (14). For the SJL strain, thymocyte precursor frequencies were estimated to be $1/11 \times 10^6$ and $1/10 \times 10^6$ for (Phe,G) and Pro--L, respectively; the relevant thymus cell frequencies for these two specificities in the DBA/1 strain were $1/19 \times 10^6$ and $1/20 \times 10^6$. No differences were found between the (Phe,G) and Pro--L thymocyte precursor frequencies within the mouse strains, the 1.9-fold differences observed between the two strains were not significant. Thus, the lack of correlation between immune response potential and the frequency of relevant thymocytes is compatible with the hypothesis that thymus cells are not involved in generating the low responses observed in poor responder mouse strains for these two specificities of (Phe,G)-Pro--L.

(Phe,G)-Pro--L contains two immunopotent regions which elicit antibodies of distinct specificities and the immune response potentials of these two regions are controlled by separate genes (6). It could therefore be argued that cellular studied using this polypeptide might involve a more complex situation than experiments in which (T,G)-Pro--L, or (Phe,G)-A--L, were investigated. Furthermore, the fact that (Phe,G)-A--L is built on a backbone of multichain poly-DL-alanine, whereas the branched polymeric side chains of (T,G)-Pro--L consist of poly-L-proline, provides an opportunity for comparing cellular aspects of genetic control of immune response as a function of the chemical structure of the immunogen. As mentioned above, a correlation was found between the immune response potentials of high and low responders and the relative numbers of splenic antigen-sensitive units stimulated. Limiting dilutions of thymocytes and bone marrow cells (as described above for (Phe,G)-Pro--L) were made for the (T,G)-Pro--L and (Phe,G)-A--L immunogens. For (T,G)-Pro--L a five-fold difference in the frequencies of relevant and limiting precursor cells was detected in the marrow of high responder SJL and low responder DBA/1 donors (see upper part of Fig. 6). Identical frequencies of thymus-derived helper cells were found in these two mouse strains (see lower part of Fig. 6). Thus, the cellular aspects of genetic regulation of immune response to (T,G)-Pro--L is similar to those found for the Pro--L immunopotent region of (Phe,G)-Pro--L (15). In contrast to the cellular studies reported for the Pro--L series of immunogens, the marrow and thymus cell dilution experiments with (Phe,G)-A--L revealed genetically associated differences in both the marrow and thymus populations of immunocytes from high (DBA/1) and low (SJL) responders (Fig. 7). In addition to a five-fold difference in limiting marrow cell precursors (similar to that seen in the Pro--L studies), a striking 12- to 40-fold difference was observed between the helper cell activity of high responder DBA/1 and low responder SJL thymocytes (15). Dilution curves of SJL thymocytes conformed to the predictions of the Poisson model, whereas those from DBA/1 donors did not (see lower part of Fig. 7). This non-Poisson curve suggests not only that there are more thymus cells relevant for generating (Phe,G)-A--L responses in the DBA/1 than in the SJL strain (compare the 5 x 10^6 - 6 x 10^7 inocula, Fig. 7), but that the helper cell activity of DBA/1 thymocytes is more efficient than that of the SJL low responder strain. The observation that the genetic defect to (Phe,G) in this strain is reflected only in the number of marrow precursors when these peptides are attached to poly-L-proline, whereas the defect is reflected in the number of both marrow and thymus immunocompetent cells when (Phe,G) is attached to poly-DL-alanine, stresses the importance of the chemical structure of the entire immunogenic macromolecule in the expression of the genetic defects for a given specificity at the cellular level.

Studies of this type are currently in progress to determine the cellular basis of genetic regulation of immune responses for the "loop"-lysozyme system. Based on the similarities observed between the synthetic polypeptide antigenic model and these natural antigens in intact SJL and DBA/1 mice (compare Tables 1 and 2), one would expect to find the cellular defect(s) for "loop"-A--L to reside both in bone marrow and thymus cells, whereas the defect for "loop"-Pro--L and for the "loop" determinant of the natural protein lysozyme should be expressed by marrow cells only.

Multiple-stranded homopolymers of ribonucleotides such as polyA-polyU have been shown to enhance the immunity of newborn and adult mice (16,17). In order to determine whether it is possible to enhance significantly low immune responses to synthetic polypeptides by polyA polyU treatment, DBA/1 and SJL mice were immunized with 10 μg (T,G)-Pro--L or (Phe,G)-A--L in complete Freund's adjuvant. Twenty-four hours later, 300 μg of polyA-polyU was administered via the tail vein. The mice were given a secondary immunization three weeks later with (T,G)-Pro--L or (Phe,G)-A--L followed by polyA-polyU. In Table 4 the results obtained after primary and secondary immunization are compared for treated and untreated high and low responder strains. Concerning (T,G)-Pro--L, the low responder DBA/1 mice injected with polyA-polyU responded as well as the untreated high responder SJL strain. An eight-fold increase in the anti-(T,G)-Pro--L titers was obtained as compared with the untreated DBA/1 animals (18). Administration of polyA-polyU to the high responder SJL strain resulted in an insignificant increase in antibody titers. No effect was observed in enhancing the low response of SJL mice to (Phe,G)-A--L by polyA-polyU treatment. Furthermore, the low response of SJL mice to (Phe,G) was not corrected by polyA-polyU treatment when this specificity was part of the (Phe,G)-Pro--L macromolecule, whereas the low Pro--L response of the DBA/1 strain was corrected using this immunogen. This contrasting influence of polyA-polyU on the low responders to the (Phe,G)

TABLE IV

ENHANCEMENT OF IMMUNE RESPONSES IN INTACT LOW RESPONDER MICE IMMUNIZED WITH SYNTHETIC POLYPEPTIDES AND INJECTED WITH polyA-polyU

Mouse Strain	Mice Injected with polyA-polyU	Range of Serum Titers[a]	
		Primary Response	Secondary Response
	Immunized and Assayed with (T,G)-Pro--L		
DBA/1	No	1:4 - 1:16	1:8 - 1:16
	Yes	1:64	1:64- 1:128
SJL	No	1:16- 1:32	1:64- 1:256
	Yes	1:16- 1:32	1:128-1:256
	Immunized and Assayed with (Phe,G)-A--L		
SJL	No	1:4	1:8 - 1:16
	Yes	1:4	1:8 - 1:16
DBA/1	No	1:16	1:128-1:512
	Yes	1:16	1:128-1:512

a - Passive hemagglutination titers based on sera from 5 - 10 individual mice.

and Pro--L determinants verifies earlier findings that different genes regulate immunological responsiveness to these specificities (6), and indicates that the phenotypic expression of these genes are functionally dissimilar.

It has been shown that the low responses of guinea pigs to hapten-polylysine conjugates were enhanced when the immunogen was complexed to acetylated bovine serum albumin (19). A similar result was obtained in low responder mice when (T,G)-A--L was complexed to methylated bovine serum albumin (MBSA) (20). Since the genetically controlled low responses to (Phe,G)-A--L and to the (Phe,G) portion of (Phe,G)-Pro--L were not enhanced by polyA-polyU, it was of interest to establish whether higher antibody titers would be obtained when low responder mice to (Phe,G)-A--L, as well as low responders to (T,G)-Pro--L, were immunized with these polypeptides complexed to MBSA. The results shown in Table 5 indicate that primary and secondary responses of DBA/1 mice to (T,G)-Pro--L were enhanced to the corresponding high responder levels. In contrast to the lack of enhancement by polyA-polyU, MBSA also increased the (Phe,G)-A--L titers in SJL mice. This enhancement was detected mainly in the secondary response, however, and titers did not reach the DBA/1 high responder levels.

The results of the experiments summarized in this paper provide an example of fundamental research aimed at better defining the role inheritance plays in immunological processes with respect to the chemical structure of the antigen and to the cell populations affected. Once the interrelationships among the genetic, molecular and cellular aspects of immunity are realized in experimental models, it may be possible to generate a strong immune response to a desired determinant (specificity) in an individual who otherwise would be a poor responder, by coupling the determinant to a macromolecule to which the individual is a high responder. The realization of this approach for characterization and modification of immunological responsiveness in humans will ultimately depend upon establishing a linkage between a given HLA type and the ability to respond to a given antigenic determinant or carrier molecule, and/or developing *in vitro* systems for screening the immune response potentials of individuals for a given immunogen. Once these techniques have been established it should be possible to combine molecular engineering of the immunogen with the genetic correlations of immune responsiveness in developing effective vaccines for human and animal use.

TABLE V

ENHANCEMENT OF IMMUNE RESPONSES IN INTACT LOW RESPONDER MICE IMMUNIZED WITH SYNTHETIC POLYPEPTIDES COMPLEXED TO METHYLATED BOVINE SERUM ALBUMIN

Mouse Strain	Immunogen Complexed With MBSA	Range of Serum Titers[a]	
		Primary Response	Secondary Response
Immunized and Assayed with (T,G)-Pro--L			
DBA/1	No	1:4 - 1:16	1:4 - 1:16
	Yes	1:64	1:128- 1:256
SJL	No	1:16- 1:32	1:32 - 1:64
	Yes	1:32- 1:64	1:32 - 1:128
Immunized and Assayed with (Phe,G)-A--L			
SJL	No	1:8 - 1:16	1:8 - 1:16
	Yes	1:16- 1:32	1:64
DBA/1	No	1:8 - 1:16	1:256
	Yes	1:16- 1:32	1:256

a - Passive hemagglutination titers based on sera from 5-10 individual mice.

REFERENCES

1. COOKE, R.A. & VANDER VEER, A. *J. Immunol.* *1:*201, 1916.
2. McDEVITT, H.O. & BODMER, W.F. *Am. J. Med.* *52:*1, 1972.
3. McDEVITT, H.O. & SELA, M. *J. Exper. Med.* *122:*517, 1965.
4. McDEVITT, H.O. & SELA, M. *J. Exper. Med.* *126:*969, 1967.
5. MOZES, E., McDEVITT, H.O., JATON, J-C. & SELA, M. *J. Exper. Med.* *130:*493, 1969.
6. MOZES, E.,McDEVITT, H.O., JATON, J-C. & SELA, M. *J. Exp. Med.* *130:*1263, 1969.
7. MOZES, E., MARON, E., ARNON, R. & SELA, M. *J. Immunol.* *106:*862, 1971.
8. SHEARER, G.M., CUDKOWICZ, G., & PRIORE, R.L. *J. Exper. Med.* *129:*185, 1969.
9. SHEARER, G.M. & CUDKOWICZ, G. *J. Exper. Med.* *129:*935, 1969.
10. NOSSAL, G.J.V., CUNNINGHAM, A., MITCHELL, G.F. & MILLER, J.F. A.P. *J. Exper. Med.* *128:*839, 1968.
11. MITCHISON, N.A. *Eur. J. Immunol.* *1:*18, 1971.
12. MOZES, E., SHEARER, G.M. & SELA, M. *J. Exper. Med.* *132:*613, 1970.
13. SHEARER, G.M., MOZES, E. & SELA, M. *J. Exper. Med.* *133:*216, 1971.
14. MOZES, E. & SHEARER, G.M. *J. Exper. Med.* *134:*141, 1971.
15. SHEARER, G.M., MOZES, E. & SELA, M. *J. Exper. Med.* *135:* 1972 (in press).
16. BRAUN, W. & NAKANO, M. *Science* *157:*819, 1967.
17. WINCHURCH, R. & BRAUN, W. *Nature* *223:*843, 1969.
18. MOZES, E., SHEARER, G.M., SELA, M. & BRAUN, W. Conversion with polynucleotides of a genetically controlled low immune response to a high response in mice immunized with a synthetic polypeptide antigen. In: Biological Effects of Polynucleotides, p. 162, R.F. Beers and W. Braun, Eds., Springer-Verlag, New York, 1970.
19. GREEN, I., PAUL, W.E. & BENACERRAF, B. *J. Exper. Med.* *123:*859, 1966.
20. McDEVITT, H.O. *J. Immunol.* *100:*485, 1968.

PERSPECTIVES IN THE CONTROL OF VIRAL DISEASES INCLUDING CANCER

Maurice R. Hilleman

Division of Virus and Cell Biology Research
Merck Institute for Therapeutic Research
West Point, Pennsylvania, U.S.A.

Among the infectious diseases, those caused by viruses stand unique in the limited benefit, if any, that can be achieved by treatment. Practical considerations demand, therefore, that primary emphasis be given to the prevention of viral infections while, at the same time, exploring all approaches that might eventually be applied to their control.

There presently are but three approaches to the specific control of viral diseases (Table 1), each with its own advantages and disadvantages. Vaccines generally provide high level immunity with long-lasting effect but are of very narrow spectrum, viz., one virus, one vaccine. The interferon mechanism, by contrast, promises broad-spectrum antiviral activity but with the disadvantage of short-term duration. Chemicals, as we now know them, posses both the disadvantages of a relatively narrow antiviral spectrum and a very short duration of effect, requiring continuous administration of the drug in order to maintain a protective effect.

CHEMOTHERAPY

The great successes which attended antibacterial chemotherapy since the start of World War II have not been paralleled for viral diseases, principally because viral metabolism is dependent upon host cellular metabolism. Presently, there are only three substances or classes of chemical substances that can be considered to be of some clinical use. These are N-methylisatin-β-thiosemicarbazone for prophylaxis of smallpox, the adamantanamines for prevention of influenza, and metabolic inhibitors such as iododeoxyuri-

TABLE I

APPROACHES TO SPECIFIC CONTROL OF VIRAL INFECTIONS

Kind	Level of Efficacy	Breadth of Protection Against Different Viruses	Duration of Protective Effect
Immunologic (Vaccines)	High	Narrow	Long
Host Resistance (Interferon and Inducers)	Moderate to high	Broad*	Short
Chemical (Drugs)	Low to moderate	Narrow	Very short

*The substance, interferon, is strongly host species-specific.

dine, cytosine arabinoside, and trifluorothymidine for treating herpes simplex of the cornea and perhaps of the central nervous system. Cognizance needs be taken, however, that there are events in viral infections in cells which are specific to the virus and which provide points against which antiviral chemicals might be directed. Increasing knowledge and sophistication in cellular and viral biochemistry should eventually permit synthesis of candidate chemicals on a directed and non-random basis. It must be noted that vaccines and interferon are preventives and that the only hope at present for cure of infection in the individual cell lies in the chemical approach. This, then, provides a real justification for continued concerted effort in chemotherapy.

INTERFERON

The broad spectrum antiviral activity shown by the interferon system has provided a basis for attempts to bring it into useful application for control of viral diseases in man and his domestic animals. The initial hope that interferon could be purified, perhaps even synthesized, and administered as an exogenous substance of prophylactic and therapeutic benefit has not been realized to date. The most serious problems relate to finding sources of interferon that will provide materials safe for use in man and to the projected high costs involved in making the substance. Added to this is the basic problem that interferon is primarily a prophylactic rather than a therapeutic substance and might not have any significant value if administered after symptoms appear. In the absence of a significant breakthrough in preparation, exogenous interferon would seem to hold little promise in human and animal medicine. Not all workers would agree with this appraisal, however, and the production and planned clinical testing of exogenous interferon is being actively pursued in a number of laboratories.

The lack of promise of exogenous interferon has led to concerted attempts to seek a suitable inducer of interferon that might be applied to cause the body to synthesize and distribute its own interferon. The search for inducers has been outstanding in two respects -- first, in the large variety of agents and substances which do induce interferon and second, in the lack of practical usefulness of these inducers because of infectivity, antigenicity, toxicity, accumulation, and the like. Of all the inducers, double-stranded ribonucleic acids alone have shown promise for clinical application and of these, the complex of polyriboinosinic and polyribocytidylic acid, commonly referred to as poly I:C, has been chosen for extensive study.

Though highly toxic for dogs and for certain rodent species, poly I:C is not highly toxic for monkeys. The markedly beneficial effects of poly I:C against acute viral infections in animals and the limited positive results obtained in tests in rodents against oncogenic viruses and transplant tumors have provided a basis for early exploratory trials in man. Trials to date in advanced cancer patients, carried out by our group with Dr. C. Young at the Sloan Kettering Institute for Cancer Research and Memorial Hospital, have not shown significant toxicity for man except for induction of fever, even when a total amount of 35 mg/kg body weight was administered intravenously during a period of 15 days. Individual doses were as high as 10 mg/kg/day. Interferon was induced or elevated in titer in 26 out of 43 (65 percent) patients tested to date, in spite of the immunologic impairment which commonly accompanies cancer.

The studies of poly I:C to date in man have been of sufficient promise to justify further investigations to determine the significance of the drug in human medicine. The greatest importance for an interferon inducer might be in the prevention of those viral infections that are caused by multiple serotypes such as the myriad types of rhinoviruses which cause the common cold and which are beyond reasonable expectation for control by vaccines. The principal deterrent to further tests in man at this time is the existence of a second biologic effect of poly I:C, that of stimulating the ordinary specific immune mechanisms as well as interferon. It has been demonstrated that poly I:C can potentiate and shorten the incubation period for a spontaneous autoimmune disease in NZB/W mice, a condition which is perhaps analogous to systemic lupus in man. At the same time, it should be noted that no antigenicity of poly I:C for man has been shown to date. Tests are presently in progress to determine safe dose levels and regimens for NZB/W mice which, once established, should permit continued cautious trials of the drug in man.

VIRAL VACCINES

One can scarcely question the remarkable effectiveness of vaccines in the prevention and control of viral diseases and the very great benefits which have resulted from their development and application. It is of some interest that the real advances in vaccine development have been sporadic and have always depended upon a major breakthrough. As shown in Table 2, the first major breakthrough in viral vaccine development was largely by serendipity -- thus Jenner's recognition of the protective effect of cowpox infection against smallpox. The second breakthrough was by sheer intellectual synthesis from ill-defined immunologic principles which led to Pasteur's rabies vaccine. From that period on, the major problem has been that of how to grow the virus. The first half of the present century saw two major breakthroughs -- the development of the embryonated hen's egg and the laboratory mouse for viral propagation. These led to yellow fever, influenza, and Japanese B encephalitis vaccines. Then came the cell culture breakthrough of the late 1940's by Enders and his associates which led to the quick development of both live and killed poliovaccines, and of adenovirus vaccine in the decade of the 1950's. With cell culture technology well established, live measles, mumps, and rubella virus vaccines were developed in the following decade. Now these vaccines are available in combined single dose formulations containing measles-mumps-rubella, measles-rubella or mumps-rubella vaccines. It is of some importance that these vaccines are against both RNA- and DNA-type viruses and include both live and killed virus vaccines. Additionally, they include both naturally attenuated (cowpox) and artificially attenuated viruses. What the future

TABLE II

DEVELOPMENT OF PRINCIPAL LICENSED VIRAL VACCINES

Time Period	Primary Breakthrough	Vaccines (Kind)
1799 - 1899	Discovery of principles	Smallpox (DNA-Live) Rabies (RNA-Killed)
1901 - 1950	Mouse and chick embryo propagation of agents	Yellow Fever (RNA-Live) Influenza A & B (RNA-Killed) Japanese B Encephalitis (RNA-Killed)
1951 - 1960	Cell culture propagation of agents	Poliomyelitis (RNA-Killed) Poliomyelitis (RNA-Live) Adenovirus (DNA-Killed)
1961 - 1970	Application of cell culture technology	Measles (RNA-Live) Mumps (RNA-Live) Rubella (RNA-Live)

holds for immunization remains to be seen but clearly some further breakthroughs will be needed. Live or killed virus vaccines against respiratory syncytial, and the parainfluenza 1, 2 and 3 viruses and Mycoplasma pneumoniae will likely be evolved and come into general use within the next decade and so afford protection against at least part of the respiratory disease spectrum. Hepatitis A and B vaccines await successful means for growing and detecting the virus in the laboratory. The herpesviruses are actively under study and the varicella-zoster complex appears to be yielding to the vaccine approach. Cytomegalovirus and infectious mononucleosis might eventually be candidates for vaccines. Trachoma vaccine success must depend upon removal of the allergic sensitizing factor from the organisms. The arboviruses are of diverse serotypes with narrow geographic distribution and must be tailored to regional needs. The great benefits of high level and long-lasting immunity that can be achieved at the present time through use of metabolizable emulsified oil adjuvant must await final determination of the significance to man of reported tumor occurrence in mice given these materials.

CANCER

The most fascinating aspect of viral research in the contemporary era, however, is the glimmer of hope that is presently being held for the prevention of some of the chronic degenerative diseases and of cancer. The concept of viral etiology in cancer in man is only a hypothesis today. It is the belief, however, that human cancer may be of infectious origin and that a virus or viruses may be a necessary and indispensable component for the induction of a portion if not all cancers in man. Though no virus of proved etiologic relationship to human cancer has been reliably propagated in the laboratory to the present time, it is on the conviction that such viruses will materialize that the development of viral vaccines will be pursued. Principal support for this belief lies in the knowledge of proved viral etiology in malignant neoplasia of rodents, cats, fowl, and frogs together with ancillary information obtained in studies of cancer in bovines, monkeys, and man. Special interest in human cancer viruses has been generated by the recent reports by Drs. Priori, McAllister, Stewart, Moore, and Sanders and their associates.

Etiology

Current research in the viral etiology of human cancer is focused on the C- and B-type viruses which are being linked with leukemia, sarcoma, and breast cancer, based mainly on the demonstration of viruses or virus-like particles in human neoplastic tissues and secretions. Similar counterparts for this are to be found in the established etiologic role of such agents in the mouse, cat, and avian leukemia-sarcoma complex and in the Bittner carcinoma of mice. Attention is also being given to the highly cell-associated group B herpesviruses which are found in association with but are of unproved relationship to Burkitt lymphoma and nasopharyngeal carcinoma and to the more ordinary herpes simplex type 2 virus which causes genital herpes, and which has been linked epidemiologically but has not been proved to cause cervical carcinoma in women. Considerable support for the general etiologic role of herpesviruses in cancer is provided in the findings on the oncogenic herpesviruses of animals which now include Marek's disease (a lymphoproliferative neoplasia of domestic chickens), Lucké renal carcinoma of frogs, cottontail rabbit lymphoma, monkey lymphoma (herpesvirus saimiri of squirrel monkeys), sheep pulmonary adenomatosis, and possibly also guinea pig leukemia, and ileocecal proliferative disease of hamsters.

If, indeed, viruses do cause human cancer and if, indeed, they can be propagated reliably in the laboratory, then what are the chances for prevention of cancer or for therapeutic treatment by means of cancer virus vaccines? A look at problems and probabilities is possible at this time.

Means of Spread

In judging the possibility for developing viral vaccines against cancer, it is necessary to consider the probable means for spread of the virus, whether it be horizontal, as in infectious disease, or vertical, as in transmission from mother to offspring either through transplacental infection or through integration in the germ plasm. There is presently one concept in vogue which states that many or perhaps all cells may carry genetic materials, called virogenes and oncogenes, that code for infectious virus and for the neoplastic transformation of cells. Though normally repressed, the virogenes and oncogenes may be derepressed by chemicals, radiation, DNA viruses, or perhaps by assistance from related RNA helper viruses, causing the cells to undergo transformation and to produce infectious transmissible virus bearing the oncogene. It is well known in animal systems that infectious oncogenic RNA-type viruses, introduced, artificially, do indeed cause cancer with high incidence that is well beyond that which occurs spontaneously, and it is possible also that these transmissible viruses may correspond to the hypothetical occult virogenes and oncogenes. The interpretation, then, is that even though cancer may arise as a spontaneous event through activation of a latent or "repository" oncogene, it might also arise as a result of a horizontally transmitted "superinfection" with an adequate dose of the corresponding virus or with yet another virus in the same animal which is already bearing the virogenes and oncogenes. Such post-natal horizontal spread seems certainly to be the principal means whereby chickens receive their tumorigenic viruses, both of RNA (leukemia) and DNA (Marek's) type. The basic question, then, is which kind of event, assuming both occur in man, is mainly responsible for cancer as it occurs in the human species. It is conceivable that either or both may occur. The recent recognition of "epidemic" occurrence of Hodgkin's disease, the evident infectious transmission of Burkitt lymphoma, and the oft noted occurrence of leukemia clusters which goes beyond the likelihood of coincidence, all give credence to the concept of transmissible infectious spread of cancer-producing agents in man. It is possible that the latent oncogene, in the practical sense, may only be the repository in nature for these viruses and the means whereby their perpetuity is guaranteed. If cancer be the result of infection with exogenous transmissible infectious virus, either as the primary oncogenic agent or as an activator, then the chances for prophylactic immunization are good. If, on the other hand, cancer is the result of activation by various means of repressed endogenous virogenes and oncogenes of inherited origin, then vaccines might have less chance to prevent the disease, primarily because infection would have been established prenatally and because immunologic control might have been (but not necessarily so) preempted, in part at least, by induction of immunologic tolerance to certain antigens of the virus.

Vaccine Development

The eventual disclosure of the etiologic factor(s) in human cancer will find the art and technology for vaccine preparation in a highly advanced state because of the progress already made with existing vaccines against acute viral diseases. Awaiting the isolation of human cancer viruses, probes can now be made using the numerous existent animal models to establish the necessary guidelines and precedents whereby human cancer virus vaccines can eventually proceed toward development. Experiments aimed at evaluating the virus vaccine approach to the control of experimental cancer in animals have been limited to date. There are, however, sufficient examples to establish the utility of the approach. One can cite very positive results obtained in immunizing against the avian leukemia-sarcoma complex, against the murine leukemia-sarcoma complex, against the adenoviruses which are oncogenic for animals, against SV_{40} and polyoma viruses, and against infectious myxoma virus of rabbits. These vaccines, in the case of RNA virus-dependent neoplasia, may even show some degree of therapeutic effect, presumably by limiting spread of the virus to new and uninfected cells within the infected host.

The most outstanding example of vaccine success, however, is the recent development of highly effective vaccines against Marek's disease of chickens. This is a lymphoproliferative neoplastic disease in chickens which causes great economic losses to the poultry industry. The disease is caused by a B-type herpesvirus and the development of the vaccine, in my judgment, is perhaps the most outstanding achievement in the virus cancer field in the last decade or two. The demonstration of an exclusively horizontal transmission of the herpesvirus which causes Marek's disease and the prevention of the disease by use of highly effective attenuated live herpesvirus vaccines presents, in my opinion, one of the best pieces of evidence against the "occult oncogene-impossible to prevent" hypothesis for cancer. The reality of live avirulent Marek's virus vaccine tends either to raise doubts as to the significance of the universal oncogene theory or to show, in the practical sense at least, that chickens, in the case of Marek's disease, may be kept alive and free of cancer by use of a herpesvirus vaccine whether the virulent virus be the primary carcinogenic agent or a cocarcinogen.

The Marek's vaccine used most commonly in the U.S.A. and in certain other countries was developed by Dr. Ben Burmester and his associates at the Regional Poultry Research Laboratory of the U.S. Department of Agriculture in East Lansing, Michigan. The vaccine consists of a naturally avirulent herpesvirus of turkeys which is grown in cell culture and is used to immunize baby chicks in their first day of life following hatching. The manner in which this vaccine works is of considerable interest, as shown in Table 3.

The fully virulent infectious virus is released from infected chickens in feather follicle cells which make up chicken dander. The virulent virus infects susceptible chicks in the environment, establishes an infection which persists for the full lifetime of the bird, and causes neoplasia with tumor production, death, and deficiencies in the conversion of carbohydrate to protein.

TABLE III

PROGRESS OF MAREK'S VIRUS INFECTION IN VACCINATED AND UNVACCINATED CHICKENS

Agent	Infection	Clinical Outcome
Virulent Marek's Herpes-virus (in chicken dander)	Persistent lifetime infection	Death, tumors, decreased egg and meat production.
Turkey Herpesvirus (avirulent vaccine - parenteral)	Persistent lifetime infection	Dual viral infection but with failure to develop clinical disease
→ Virulent Marek's Herpesvirus (in chicken dander)	Persistent lifetime infection	

The avirulent turkey herpesvirus vaccine is given to chicks at one day of age, and, like virulent virus, it also establishes a virus infection that persists for the lifetime of the bird but it differs in that it does not cause clinical disease. Importantly, this avirulent virus does not prevent subsequent infection with the fully virulent Marek's virus. What the prior infection with avirulent virus does is to prevent the expression of the virulent virus as clinical neoplasia. This immunity against the development of cancer appears to reside either in some ill-defined biological antagonism between vaccine virus-infected cells and virulent virus-infected cells (e.g., interferon or intrinsic interference) or, perhaps, in the retention of a degree of immunologic normalcy of the lymphoid cellular immune mechanisms. It is known that infection with Marek's disease virus does affect both the bursal and thymic lymphoid systems in chickens with reported depression of both humoral and cellular immune responses. A complementary finding is provided by the observation in some but not all trials of Marek's vaccine that there can be reduction in deaths due to causes other than definable Marek's disease. Assuming validity of the findings, such evidence is consistent with retention of a functional immune system that can cope with a variety of life-limiting disease agents.

There are at least two important lessons to be learned from the Marek's vaccine, I believe. First is the lesson that a vaccine need not prevent infection with virulent virus in order to prevent cancer. Instead, it needs only to limit the ability of the virulent virus to express itself clinically as cancer. Second, there is an alert to the need for search for avirulent counterparts of human oncogenic viruses and it is possible that these might be bountifully distributed in nature. It is worthy of note that Barski and his associates have described a nonleukemogenic C-type murine virus which interferes with induction of neoplasia by Gross leukemia virus.

It is also worthy of special note that Marek's disease vaccine for chickens represents the first and only effective vaccine for the control of a naturally occurring malignant neoplasia in any species, and it is reasonable that special attention be given to its development, since it may provide guidelines for human cancer vaccines, especially for Burkitt lymphoma and for nasopharyngeal carcinoma which appear to be caused by herpesviruses of the same general group. It is well established that scientific findings are not isolated events and that what is known about one virus or virus-host system can often be applied to another. This is certainly true in the field of comparative oncology and it may be worthy of emphasis that the foundations of modern knowledge of mammalian RNA leukemia and sarcoma viruses are based on the previous work done with chicken viruses. It is almost a certainty, also, that further progress with oncogenic mammalian herpesviruses will have its foundation in the advances which have been made with Marek's disease.

Hurdles to Cross

The approach to the control of cancer by vaccines in man is clearly in the prenatal stage of development and cannot proceed in the final sense until the etiologically valid human oncogenic viruses are reliably propagated in the laboratory. It is not too early, however, to seek guidelines and to establish new precedents in properly designed animal experiments which will pave the way for experimental use of vaccines in man, once the causative viruses are adequately available for use. Certainly, many of the concepts and precedents held sacred up to now in the preparation and use of vaccines against acute viral diseases will need be altered to accommodate vaccines against cancer. It seems likely as of now that cancer virus itself will need to be used in the viral vaccine, in killed or attenuated form, and that virus derived from serially passaged "shedder" cultures will provide the most practical source. Obviously, the discovery of naturally avirulent variants of important oncogenic viruses (the equivalent perhaps of naturally avirulent Marek's virus of chickens as employed by Rispen to make vaccine) might go far toward precluding the problem of oncogenicity in the first place since application of non-oncogenic viruses should pose no question of safety. Additionally, the development of animal host systems more sensitive to neoplasia than man himself would greatly simplify the problem of establishing the safety of attenuated live virus vaccines. The use of subunit viral vaccines free of viral nucleic acid might also prove more acceptable than whole virus, even though inactivated.

Equally difficult to establishing safety is the matter of determining protective efficacy, especially if more than one virus causes cancer, or if the vaccine is less than 100 percent effective, or the incubation period is very long. This situation might be considerably simplified if the oncogenic virus produced clinically recognizable acute infectious disease as well as cancer, as e.g., if Burkitt lymphoma E-B virus causes infectious mononucleosis as well as cancer. Proved protective efficacy of a vaccine against such acute infectious disease might then be extrapolated to indicate protection against neoplasia as well. Making cancer a notifiable disease with compulsory autopsy and the establishment of national cancer registries could greatly facilitate all studies of cancer epidemiology and prevention. Without an adequate surveillance system, evaluation of vaccines against clinical cancer would be clearly impossible.

Concluding Remarks

In conclusion, it can scarcely be argued that the role of viruses in cancer and the prevention of cancer by viral vaccines is an immensely complex situation which is only in its earliest stages of exploration. The task seems enormous but is clearly justifiable considering that approximately 1/4 of all persons develop cancer and 1/5 die of it. The cancer situation could become exaggerated if environmental or other factors should increase the incidence of cancer at a lower age, such as has occurred for Marek's disease in chicken flocks.

No quick solution to the cancer problem can be expected and no safe and effective vaccine can be expected within a short period of time. Such developments might best be reckoned in decades rather than years. It seems a necessary requirement that there will need to be a reevaluation and realignment of present concepts of risk vs. benefit in the application of cancer virus vaccines, to less rigorous requirements than now exist, since the disease we are considering carries a guaranteed mortality rate of 80 percent for those afflicted.

Whatever the wish, precedent and caution will prevail and it will be necessary, in the practical sense, to apply the most stringent inherent safety criteria and made the least radical departure from established precedent in initiating studies in man. To this end, killed virus or subunit vaccines, or naturally avirulent live virus vaccines, offer the greatest chance for acceptance and should probably be applied initially to attempt prevention or limitation of neoplastic expression of existent infection or disease.

ACKNOWLEDGEMENT

Work on cancer in our laboratories is supported under Contract No. NIH-71-2059 within the Special Virus Cancer Program of the National Cancer Institute, National Institutes of Health, U.S. Public Health Service.

PRODUCTION OF VACCINES WITH SPECIAL REFERENCE TO RUBELLA VACCINE RA 27/3 STRAIN IN WI 38 CELLS

A. J. Beale

Biological Division
The Wellcome Research Laboratories
Beckenham, Kent, U.K.

When a disease is sufficiently serious to warrant prevention and a vaccine has been seen to be technically possible, it is necessary to devise methods of preparation and testing that minimize the dangers inherent in large scale manufacture. It is one thing for an investigator to prepare a few doses of vaccine with loving care in his laboratory to demonstrate its potential usefulness and quite another to prepare millions of doses of a safe and effective vaccine, year by year. The methods for controlling industrial production of vaccines have been developed slowly through the years and are still being developed. There have been some spectacular errors, some of which are listed in Table 1, but on the whole the record has been one of solid progress. Indeed the very success of vaccination programs has led to new problems for public health officials. Thus the control of smallpox, largely by vaccine, has brought a new balance of risks of vaccination against the risks of the disease. Because the risks of complications of vaccination now outweigh the risks of smallpox, many countries are abandoning routine smallpox vaccine, and as other diseases come under control the use of other vaccines may be brought into question.

With regard to large-scale vaccine production it soon became apparent, notably at the time of the Lubeck disaster, that a prime essential is to have a recognized expert in sole charge. The authorities in most countries have insisted that this approved expert or responsible head is the final professional authority responsible for the quality of the product and,in the event of disaster, cannot excuse himself by saying the President or Managing Director or whatever the boss is called, told him that profits were

TABLE I

FAULTS IN THE PREPARATION OF VACCINES

Fault	Example
1. Use of virulent strain instead of attenuated	Lubeck 1929 KIEL strain used instead of BCG. (207 cases - 72 deaths)
2. Failure to use seed lot system	17D yellow fever produced encephalitis in Brazil in 1941. New seed made. (199 cases - 1 death)
3. Failure of inactivation	Residual poliovirus in killed poliovaccine "cutter" incident U.S.A. 1955. (260 cases - 10 deaths)
4. Contamination by extraneous agents	Yellow fever vaccine contaminated with serum hepatitis virus in serum used as stabilizer, U.S.A., 1942. (28,585 cases - 62 deaths)
5. Inherent danger unsatisfactory seed strain	Lederle-Cox strains of attenuated poliovirus.

more important. Ultimately, it is this expert who goes to prison, as did Dr. Deyke after the Lubeck disaster, if negligence is proved.

The need for the whole apparatus of an expert staff for manufacturing and testing and the idea of rigid segregation of production staff and areas was thus gradually built up, first for anaerobic spore-bearing organisms but subsequently reinforced for living attenuated virus vaccines. Inspection of premises to see that there were adequate safeguards against contamination was also introduced. All the stages of manufacture of a living vaccine must be segregated. In addition, for killed vaccines it is necessary to separate those stages associated with living virus from those associated with killed virus and satisfactory methods have evolved and proved effective for the manufacture of killed vaccines, for example against poliomyelitis and influenza in man, Newcastle disease, foot and mouth disease and canine hepatitis in animals.

The quality of a vaccine is critically dependent on the seed used to produce it. Successive subcultivation or passage of bacteria and viruses in the laboratory leads to modifications in antigenic structure, or loss of virulence, or both. This led, for bacterial vaccines, to insistence on the use of freshly isolated strains, and also to establishment of the seed system, as soon as it became possible to store stocks of seed for years at low temperature or by freeze-drying. In this way seed of reproducible quality is assured; it can be exhaustively tested for extraneous agents and maintained without risk of contamination. The quality of vaccine made from this seed can be tested in the laboratory and in the field for efficacy and safety. It is now universally accepted that a seed lot system is essential for efficient vaccine manufacture, especially for attenuated virus vaccines, but indeed also for killed vaccines. The preparation and testing of vaccine seeds is however not always possible - for example with influenza. Antigenic variants arise and the preparation of vaccine is an urgent matter. The use of genetic recombination would probably permit seed capable of yielding large amounts of killed vaccine to be manufactured specially. Living influenza vaccines might also be made in this way, but the need for adequate testing of the seed in the laboratory and in man almost certainly implies that only killed vaccines can be made in time to counter an epidemic.

Viruses have to be produced in living cells and initially this involved the use of intact animals for virus propagation, thus involving the hazards of introducing extraneous agents from the host animals and of contamination of the vaccine with host tissues. Despite these disadvantages, both of which are serious, smallpox, rabies and yellow fever vaccines are all still sometimes made in this way. Most vaccines nowadays, however, are made in eggs or cell cultures, giving virus in greater yield and of higher purity. Yellow fever vaccine is the most important living vaccine now made in avian leucosis-free eggs, and it represents a considerable improvement on vaccines made from animal tissue. Killed rabies and influenza vaccines are made in duck and chick embryo. These vaccines still contain appreciable quantities of host cell protein which may give rise to allergic reactions. Technological advances, notably zonal centrifugation and virus splitting, have enabled much purer virus to be prepared and this has been extensively applied to killed influenza vaccine. Shortly we will be able to evaluate vaccines based on purified haemagglution and neuraminidase.

Cell culture was first applied widely to the manufacture of poliovaccine, first the killed and subsequently the living attenuated virus. It was soon realized that the monkey kidney cells used were frequently contaminated with viruses which were more or less easy to detect and the need to find an alternative cell substrate for poliovaccine became apparent. Other vaccines have been made in duck embryo or chick embryo fibroblasts and in dog and rabbit kidney cells. The animals providing these tissues, unlike monkeys, can be conveniently maintained in enclosed colonies which minimize the risks of contamination by extraneous agents. There would, however, be obvious merits in applying the seed lot system to the cell substrate as well as to the virus, for the same reasons, to ensure consistent quality of the substrate and further minimize the dangers of contamination by extraneous agents.

So far, only one cell substrate that can be used as a cell seed basis, the human diploid cell strain WI 38, has been extensively tested for the presence of extraneous agents. The techniques employed have involved extensive tests in tissue cultures and animals: fluorescent antibody staining tests: electron microscopy, involving sectioning of cells and disruption and negative staining with phosphotungstic acid: light microscopy of cells, both fresh and stained: karyological examination: determination of antigenic composition, and of growth characteristics and susceptibility to viruses. None of these techniques has revealed any extraneous virus present in WI 38 cells, while they have proved capable of detecting viral and mycoplasma infections that were introduced subsequently into the cells. Since it is never possible to prove a negative in a formal sense, doubts have remained. As Pasteur observed in connection with spontaneous generation, all you can hope to do is to demonstrate the fallacies of contrary experiments. The reservations about WI 38 cells are not based on experimental findings; these doubts were concerned first with the possibility that they may contain hepatitis viruses. It is now quite clear they are free from this contamination; no evidence has been obtained for the presence of Australia antigen either by electron microscopy or serology. Moreover, careful follow-up has shown that extensive use of vaccines prepared on WI 38 cells has not been followed by hepatitis, whereas contamination of other vaccines in the past with hepatitis virus was readily detected. A second doubt concerns the presence of an agent capable of causing human malignant disease in the cells. No agent has been demonstrated or isolated, nor do the cells show any tumorigenic properties in immunosuppressed hamsters or mice. Study of known oncogenic viruses shows that they are more likely to cause tumors in unnatural hosts than in the natural one. For example, SV40 produces tumors in hamsters, not in monkeys; and adenoviruses also cause tumors in hamsters, but there is no evidence that they do so in man. Also, RNA tumor viruses cross species boundaries and when they do so, this is more a property of the virus strain than the genetic constitution of the host. For example the Schmidt Ruppin strain of Rous sarcoma virus causes tumors in many species of mammals, including monkeys as well as chickens.

In order to demonstrate the oncogenicity of RNA tumor viruses in the host animals it is necessary not only to use especially genetically susceptible inbred lines but also to ensure that they lack antibody to the virus. In theory, primary cells as well as WI 38 cells may be contaminated with hypothetical oncogenic viruses: if they are so, the dangers from viruses in primary non-human cells is probably at least as great or greater than from WI 38 cells because of the ability of oncogenic viruses to cross species barriers and because each time a new primary culture is produced, there is an unknown and new risk of such an event.

Recently the ability to induce the appearance of 'C' particles in otherwise normal cells, for example by exposure to iododeoxyuridine, and the promulgation of the oncogene theory suggest that WI 38 cells, in common with all other cells, may contain this gene. However, since the oncogene is postulated to be universal to all cells, this does not give the use of primary cells any advantage over the use of WI 38 cells. The absence of C particles in WI 38 cells or in primary cells used for vaccine production implies at least that they are not switched on for tumor virus production. Another doubt about the use of WI 38 cells has been the possibility that they may induce immunity to HLA histocompatability antigens in the recipients of vaccine. The cells are typed in the HLA system as having a major HLA 2 antigen. Studies carried out by Dr. Sanderson at Queen Victoria Hospital, East Grinstead, have shown no detectable antigen in Rubella vaccine RA 27/3, nor in poliovaccine prepared on WI 38 cells. Moreover, HLA sensitization occurs naturally in women from the fetus and any hypothetical response to a vaccine prepared in WI 38 cells is not likely to be important against this background stimulation.

The vaccines that have been made on WI 38 cells are shown in Table 2.

Rubella vaccine RA 27/3, developed by Plotkin, has been used at the Wellcome Research Laboratories to prepare vaccine in WI 38 cells using a seed lot system. The major contamination hazards that remain in this system are the trypsin, the serum, and the handling of the cultures to build up the cell stock. Large scale testing of the reagents before they are used in production is at present the only available safeguard. It has been shown that calf

TABLE II

VACCINES PREPARED ON WI 38 CELLS

Vaccines	Type	Country	Licensing Status
Poliomyelitis	O.P.V.	Yugoslavia U.K. U.S.A.	Licensed Licensed License applied for
Rubella	Living parenteral	Yugoslavia U.K. France	Licensed Licensed Licensed
	Intranasal		Experimental
Adenovirus	Living oral	U.S.A.	Experimental
	Killed subunit		Experimental
Measles	Living parenteral	Yugoslavia U.S.S.R.	Licensed Licensed
Rhinovirus	Killed parenteral	U.K. U.S.A.	Experimental Experimental

serum can be contaminated with viruses, notably reovirus, bovine diarrhoea, infectious bovine rhinotracheitis and para-influenza; as well as mycoplasma and bacteria. All of these contaminants can be excluded by suitable tests. Future research will surely find a substitute for serum.

The system of production we have employed for the production of rubella vaccine in WI 38 cells is shown in Table 3. The RA 27/3 strain of rubella vaccine has distinctive characteristics which are listed in Table 4. These characteristics on the one hand enable the strain to be recognized in the laboratory and, on the other, suggest that the strain may provide a better quality and confer a

TABLE III

SCHEME FOR PRODUCTION OF WI 38 CELLS FOR VACCINE PRODUCTION

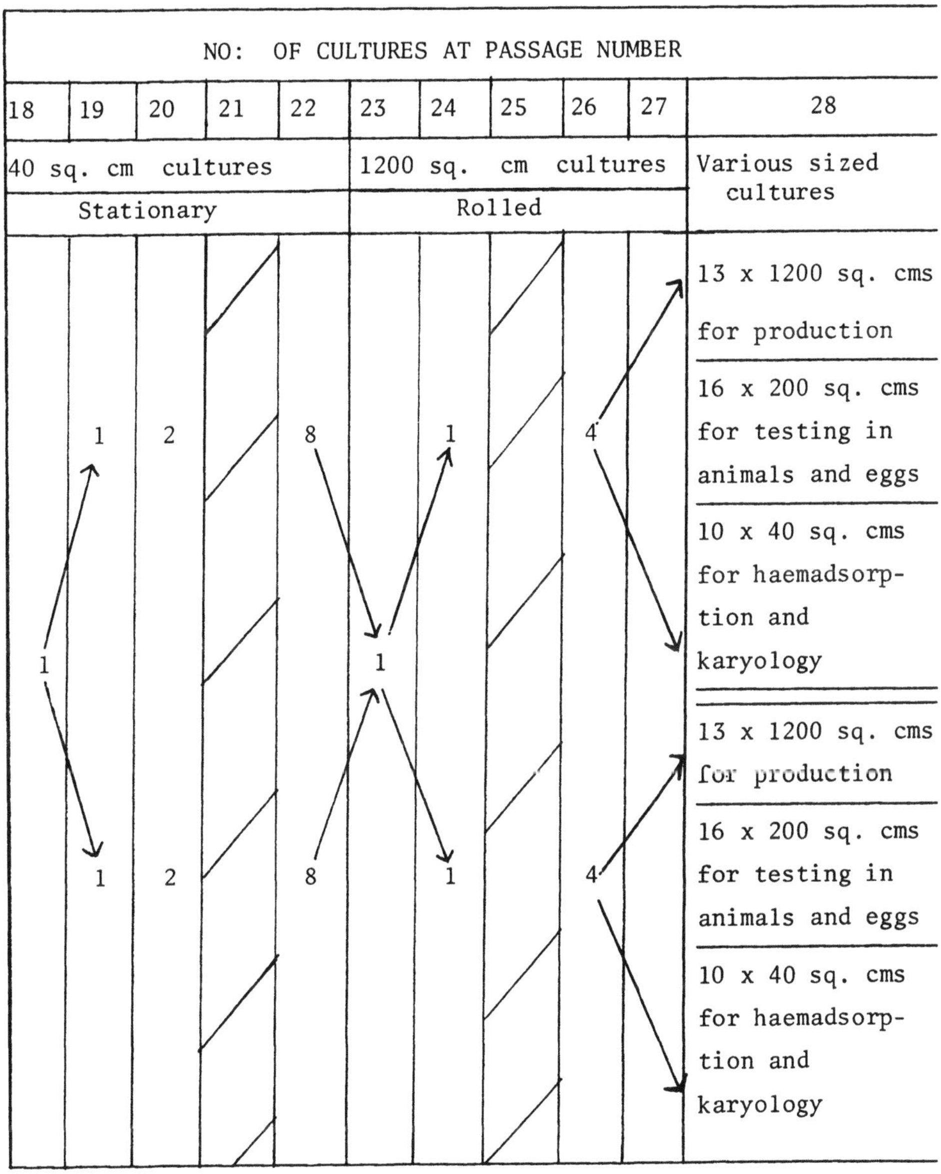

NO: OF CULTURES AT PASSAGE NUMBER										
18	19	20	21	22	23	24	25	26	27	28
40 sq. cm cultures					1200 sq. cm cultures					Various sized cultures
Stationary					Rolled					
										13 x 1200 sq. cms for production
	1	2		8		1		4		16 x 200 sq. cms for testing in animals and eggs
										10 x 40 sq. cms for haemadsorption and karyology
1					1					
										13 x 1200 sq. cms for production
	1	2		8		1		4		16 x 200 sq. cms for testing in animals and eggs
										10 x 40 sq. cms for haemadsorption and karyology

TABLE IV

CHARACTERISTICS OF RA 27/3 STRAIN RUBELLA VACCINE

1. Typical plaque morphology.
2. Infects intranasally as well as subcutaneously.
3. Produces secretory IgA antibodies in respiratory tract.
4. Produces iota and theta antibodies.
5. Boosts vaccine antibody levels when given intranasally.
6. Produces similar degree of resistance to reinfection as natural disease.

longer lasting immunity on man. The particular properties of the strain in relationship to reinfection in the respiratory tract, a characteristic similar to that of oral poliovaccine, make it particularly valuable for those countries where the public health authorities wish to eradicate the disease by community programs.

PREPARATION OF VACCINES - CELL SUBSTRATES

Frank T. Perkins

National Institute for Medical Research

London, England

Since the time it was discovered that viruses would replicate in cell cultures grown *in vitro*, techniques for the propagation of cells and improvement of virus yields have been undergoing modifications.

Fifty years ago the only three viral vaccines used were prepared in or on living animals or birds. Smallpox virus was grown on the skin of animals and the vaccine made from the lymph scraped from the infected tissues. Rabies virus was grown in the brains of susceptible animals and the vaccine consisted of the brain tissue containing the virus which was killed by phenol. Yellow fever virus was grown in fertile eggs from hens and the vaccine made from the infected embryos. At that time, few tests were done on the animals or eggs used in the production of these vaccines and indeed little was known about the viruses either infecting or inherently endemic in the birds and animals.

Virology as we know it today, especially with respect to vaccine production, really started about sixteen years ago. When a vaccine against poliomyelitis was urgently required, there was no known easily available susceptible laboratory animal and the production of this vaccine had to await further technical developments. Two major advances made at about the same time had the most profound effects on the production of viruses on a large scale. Enders, Robbins and Weller (1) placed the growth of cell cultures *in vitro* on a firm footing and showed that poliomyelitis virus could be grown in tissue culture on a commercial scale. This was indeed a significant development, but it would not have had such a potentially universal application had not penicillin, discovered by Fleming, Chain and Florey, been so successful in suppressing the bacterial contaminants that had bedevilled tissue culture for so many years. The tissue chosen for poliomyelitis vaccine production was grown from monkey kidneys and the eradication of the disease in many countries is now history. As a result of the opening of new frontiers in virology by the use of tissue culture, not only has the presence of hitherto undetected viruses been revealed, but also effects of both virus/cell and virus/virus interactions. There have been as many as 58 simian viruses identified so far, several of which occur as frequent contaminants of monkey kidney tissues. Today, we demand the use of a virus-free substrate so that there will be no possibility of interaction with the vaccine virus.

The current trend has been to use cell cultures prepared from the tissue of clean animals or birds. Thus, measles virus is grown in chick cell fibroblasts derived from the fertile eggs of chickens known by continuous monitoring to be free from the presence of fowl leucosis viruses. Rubella vaccine is currently being prepared in cell cultures grown from dog kidneys, rabbit kidneys or duck embryos.

There have been many years of experience in the growth of rabbit kidney cell cultures and it is interesting to note that few viruses have been isolated from rabbits bred in the laboratory. When the progeny are produced from dams shown to be free from antibodies to rabbit viruses and thereafter bred in a clean environment and closed colony, the ideal has been almost achieved. Cell cultures prepared under these conditions from more than 700 pairs of rabbit kidneys were shown by an extensive series of tests to be free from all viruses.

Similar results have been observed also when a closed colony of carefully screened ducks is established and the eggs produced under such ideal conditions. These measures have contributed tremendously to the safety of vaccines, but although they should be encouraged, they cannot be regarded as the ultimate answer.

When we look at the huge developments that have taken place in virus vaccine production, it is surprising that so little attention has been given to standardization of the cell substrate. There is a wealth of information on the growth requirements of different cell cultures and, as far as we are able, most cell cultures today are grown in media the composition of which is carefully controlled. The most variable constituent of culture media is calf serum and there is much research today into the important constituent in the serum supplying the growth requirements. The recent finding, by Barile and Kern (2) of the National Institute of Health, U.S.A., that more than half the lots of calf serum available through commercial sources are contaminated with mycoplasma begins to explain why so many cells in continuous propagation become contaminated. The virus used for vaccine production is selected with the utmost caution, after carefully controlled clinical trials to ensure that it is both safe and immunogenic. Indeed, the virus seed pool used as the starting point for the production of each batch of vaccine is thoroughly checked to ensure its freedom from extraneous agents and untoward characteristics. Finally, each batch of vaccine undergoes the most stringent tests to ensure its safety. It seems logical, therefore, to suggest that just as much care and attention should be given to the selection, testing and standardization of the cell substrate used for the propagation of the virus used for vaccine production.

What are the alternatives to primary monkey or kidney tissue? Several have been suggested: Earle's mouse L cells, continuous monkey and rabbit kidney cells and even chick embryo fibroblast cell lines; in making a choice several criteria must be satisfied.

1. The cell must remain normal throughout life.

2. It should be embryonic tissue, since this is the least likely to be inherently contaminated.

3. It should be tissue from a non-differentiating organ.

4. The tissue must undergo a sufficient number of doublings to provide an economic source for the manufacturer.

5. It should be a tissue susceptible to most human viruses.

Such a cell line was started by Dr. L. Hayflick, when at the Wistar Institute, and Dr. P. Moorhead (3); they established a population of human embryo lung fibroblast cells, one such cell strain being known as WI 38. Many laboratories have examined this tissue during the last ten years and none has found a contaminating virus, whereas all have found the cells to remain normal throughout 30 to 35 cell doublings. We have learnt a great deal about the practical limits of handling such cells and we are now in a position to propose recommendations to those wishing to establish their own cell line.

In general, the criteria are concerned with obtaining uncontaminated tissue from a normal person, verifying its normality throughout its finite life and showing that there are not likely to be extraneous agents, or untoward reactions occurring in use. Many of the tests may seem somewhat tedious but there are no tests proposed for a new cell substrate that have not been satisfied already by the WI 38 strain.

HISTORY AND GENEALOGY OF THE CELL STRAIN

It is most important to know the history of the cell strain and the data required include the age and sex of the donor. Hayflick started with fetal tissue because this was most likely to be free from contaminants. The possibility of the presence of extraneous agents would be much reduced by the placental barrier and taking the fetus by caesarian section would still further prevent contamination by external sources. Hayflick also comments that he purposely chose non-functional cells and avoided the use of kidney because of its likelihood of being a reservoir for latent viruses. This reduced the choice to skin, muscle, lung, etc. and the choice of lung in the case of WI 38 was arbitrary, save that it was an internal organ protected from contamination by the external skeleton. Knowledge of the sex of the donor is required merely to act as a marker in the event of cross contamination of the cell line, since the sex chromosome can be detected so easily; however, it is perhaps needed more for the sake of complete documentation than for any operational reason. Where applicable, it is important to have a full and detailed family history of the donor, particularly with respect to congenital abnormalities or genetic defects, presence or absence of evidence of neoplastic disease in the donor, parents and living siblings at the time the cell strain is established. It is appreciated that these data are particularly applicable for the establishment of a human cell strain, but even if an animal cell strain is being considered it is essential to have an accurate record of the health of the stock.

Finally, it is necessary to have a full record of the cultural history of the cell strain, including the method used to establish the initial outgrowth of cells from the tissue pieces.

CULTURE MEDIA

There are many culture media used for cell growth, some of which are more toxic than others. Parker (4), Eagle (5), and others have all proposed satisfactory balanced salt solutions and when these are added to amino acids, vitamins, nucleotides and serum, a complete medium is obtained. The medium used for the initial outgrowth of the cells from the tissue pieces is best for the continued propagation of the cells. For this reason, it is important that an accurate description of the medium composition be recorded, since a sudden change of medium during propagation may cause chromosome abnormalities. It is also important to have a large batch of fully tested serum in stock, since deficiencies or toxicities of serum may also cause changes in the karyology. We do not regard a serum as being fully tested until it has been used to support the growth of the cells for at least five cell doublings.

GROWTH CHARACTERISTICS

The time taken for cell doublings, as well as the number of doublings occurring in the finite life of the cell, are critical characteristics. Infection of the cells most often destroys them, but may cause them to grow more slowly. Furthermore, transformation of the cell may occur by infection with an oncogenic virus and although this may not cause a change in cell doubling time, it will certainly give the cell indefinite life. Both these parameters, therefore, are good markers.

FREEZING OF CELL SEED

The greatest advantage in the use of a cell strain for virus production is the facility to freeze the cell population indefinitely in small aliquots until such time as a sample has been exhaustively examined and the cell population shown to be free from extraneous agents and untoward reactions. It is important to freeze and thaw the cells in such a manner that the greatest number survive both the freezing cycle and the thawing process. During the freezing cycle, the cells are protected from damage by the use of glycerol or dimethyl sulphoxide $(CH_3)_2.SO$. There are no significant advantages of one over the other, but we do find that with DMSO there is a higher survival rate of cells.

The cells must be cooled for the first 20° to 30°C at a rate of 1°C per minute, after which they may be reduced quickly to a very low temperature. The highest temperature at which they should be stored is -70°C, but they can be preserved for much longer periods in either liquid nitrogen (-190°C) or in the gas phase of a liquid nitrogen container. Certainly, the half life of cells is significantly decreased by every degree above -70°C, until at -50°C the half life is as short as three weeks.

As much attention should be paid to the thawing of the cells as to the freezing. Cells frozen in ampoules in liquid nitrogen should be handled with care; a face vizor must be used in case the ampoules explode. As soon as it is removed from the liquid nitrogen, the ampoule should be immersed in warm alcohol and thawed rapidly. Alcohol is used so that the outside of the ampoule will remain sterile and no contamination will occur during transfer of the thawed cells to a growth bottle.

KARYOLOGY

At the onset it should be made clear that a normal karyology does not necessarily free a tissue from having untoward properties. The importance of monitoring cells by karyological studies, however, is to show that there have been no dramatic changes during propagation. The sampling of cells for such studies is a compromise between the ideal and the practical. These examinations are extremely time-consuming and tedious; a fully trained karyologist has to spend many hours at this routine work and much thought has been put into selecting the cell sample so that a reliable answer as to the normality of the cells will be obtained without an excessive amount of work.

A certain amount of discrepance between findings from different laboratories has arisen, as a result of using different criteria for abnormalities. Criteria of acceptability for the various analyses are shown in Table 1. The limits of acceptability have been selected as a result of many years of observation -- it is known that the WI 38 cells, for example, can meet these requirements. It is worth emphasizing that the suggested limits of abnormality above which the cell substrate should be rejected are based on frequencies of abnormality that may occur. Thus the required criteria are merely a sensitive probe that the cell has remained normal throughout propagation.

TESTS FOR FREEDOM FROM ADVENTITIOUS AGENTS

It is understandable that any new cell substrate suggested for use on a large scale must be thoroughly checked for the presence of adventitious agents. Thus any system uniquely capable of detecting a particular contaminant must be included in the multiple tests.

Table 2 summarizes the tests applied today in order to have a complete cover of known bacteria, fungi, mycoplasma and viruses.

HETEROTRANSPLANT STUDIES

One of the greatest difficulties in obtaining approval for a new cell substrate is the challenge that it may carry a cancer factor. The critics have not been able to explain what this is, but for practical purposes it is an unanswerable criticism since many thousands of vaccinees would have to remain under surveillance for many years before the critics would be satisfied. In view of the known high incidence of contaminants in some cell substrates, however, particularly monkey kidney, a fully characterized and noncontaminated cell substrate would be an enormous step forward in spite of our inability to answer the critics fully on this point.

TABLE I

CRITERIA OF ACCEPTABILITY BASED ON KARYOLOGICAL ANALYSES

Examination	No. of Cells Taken	Observations
1. Exact counts	100 metaphase cells	$\not>$ 2% 2n + 1 + 2 or + 3 etc., not acceptable.
2. Analysis of karyotype	one of the above cells in (1)	Photographic reconstruction to show cells are human.
3. Chromosome breaks and gaps	100 cells in (1)	Breaks may occur in one or both arms of the chromosome and they are included if they are a gap wider than the arm in which they occur. These should be $\not>$ 8%.
4. Structural chromosomal abnormalities	100 cells in (1)	Unstable structural abnormalities (dicentrics, rings, exchange configura tion, quadriradials, etc.). Stable structural abnormalities (deletions, inversions, reciprocal translocations). These should not exceed 1%.
5. Polyploidy	300 unselected metaphase cells	There should not be more than 15 polyploid cells in the 300 examined.

TABLE II

TESTS FOR FREEDOM FROM ADVENTITIOUS AGENTS

The tests used to detect the possibility that a new cell substrate harbors an adventitious agent are multiple.

1. Direct observation.
2. Inoculation of media for the detection of bacteria, fungi and mycoplasma.
3. Inoculation of cell cultures of HEK, MK, RK, Human cell line (HeLa) for the detection of viruses.
4. Inoculation of laboratory animals, embryonated eggs, s/c, i/c in newborn hamsters, i/c into suckling mice, adult mice, guinea pigs and rabbits.

A test that is available to us is inoculation into the hamster cheek pouch to observe whether cells establish and develop into a tumor. Here again, there is no absolute correlation between inability to establish a tumor in the cheek pouch and safety for man, but if a tumor is established then the cell substrate cannot be considered for further use.

It must be emphasized that this is a relatively insensitive test and we have made laboratory animals (mice) more sensitive to the inoculation of foreign cells by treating them with antilymphocyte globulin (Stanbridge and Perkins (8)). Already we have obtained large tumors in mice by inoculating HeLa cells, which are rapidly rejected by an untreated mouse. These tests are proving most useful in testing a new cell substrate.

SPECIES SPECIFICITY

It seems almost superfluous to suggest that a species specificity test must be included. The most important information which is obtained from this test is verification that the cell population is homogeneous and has not become contaminated with another cell curing the establishment of the frozen reserve of cells. There seems little to choose between the four tests available.

Cell substrates must be registered with the appropriate licensing authority with results of all tests before they may be considered as substrates for virus vaccine production.

The availability of specific antisera for the purpose of typing tissue antigens has made possible the "fingerprinting" of human diploid cell populations. Such characterization should be included in order that any accidental cross contamination which may occur later can be detected.

All the tests we have been considering are those applied to a new cell substrate to establish its suitability for virus vaccine production. When it has been approved, additional tests must be made on the particular batch of tissue used, to ensure freedom from contamination or abnormality, as well as tests on the virus harvest. The advantage of using a standardized cell substrate therefore is not in reducing work but in making vaccines safer by knowing a clean substrate has been used. It is also of enormous economic importance to the vaccine manufacturer to know that the discard of a contaminated virus pool or substrate will be a rare event rather than the frequent disappointment that it has been in the past.

THE FUTURE OF A STANDARDIZED CELL SUBSTRATE

In Yugoslavia, for the last five years poliomyelitis vaccine (oral) has been produced on human embryo lung fibroblast (WI 38) cultures and for the last three years measles vaccine produced on these cells has been administered by the parenteral route. These vaccines have been given to many thousands of children without untoward reactions.

In the United Kingdom, the first vaccine to be produced (and licensed for sale) on WI 38 cells was rubella vaccine which is given by the parenteral route to young adults. Poliomyelitis vaccine (oral) made on this cell substrate has also been licensed and we shall soon stop using vaccines made in monkey kidney cell cultures.

There is an explosion of activity in the use of diploid cell cultures and it is anticipated that the U.S.A. will license vaccines made on WI 38 cells this year. There is also much work in progress in America to attempt to establish diploid cell cultures from animal species, in particular the rabbit and monkey. It should not be forgotten, however, that many years of intensive investigation of the WI 38 cells preceded its use for vaccine production. Although some success has been achieved in the production of rabbit and monkey diploid cell populations there is still much to be done to prove that these lines are stable, retain their normal karyology throughout their life and that none of the lines has undergone spontaneous transformation.

Whatever the outcome of these newer diploid cell populations, it appears certain that the future production of virus vaccines will be based on standardized, fully characterized diploid cell populations. Today the WI 38 cells and MRC-5 cell strains (another human embryo lung fibroblast) are the only available substrates that have satisfied all the stringent requirements.

REFERENCES

1. ENDERS, J.F., WELLER, T.H. & ROBBINS, F.C. *Science 109*:85, 1949.
2. BARILE, M.F. & KERN, J. *Proc. Soc. Exper. Biol. Med. 138*: 432, 1971.
3. HAYFLICK, L. & MOORHEAD, P.S. *Exper. Cell Res. 25*:585, 1961.
4. MORGAN, J.F., MORTON, H.J. & PARKER, R.C. *Proc. Soc. Exper. Biol. Med. 73*:1, 1950.
5. EAGLE, H. *Science 130*:432, 1959.
6. PUCK, T.T., CIECIURA, STEVEN J. & ROBINSON, A. *J. Exper. Med. 108*:945, 1958.
7. LEIBOVITZ, A. *Am. J. Hyg. 78*:173, 1963.
8. STANBRIDGE, E. & PERKINS, F.T. *Nature 221*:80, 1969.

VIRAL VACCINES: VARIOUS CELL SUBSTRATES AND LONG-TERM PROSPECTIVE STUDIES

Ruth L. Kirschstein and John C. Petricciani
Laboratory of Pathology, Division of Biologics Standards, National Institutes of Health
U.S. Public Health Service, Department of Health, Education and Welfare, Bethesda, Maryland, U.S.A.

We will attempt to give an overview of the developments in the use of various cell substrates for the production of viral vaccines that has led to the present thinking of the regulatory agency of the United States, the Division of Biologics Standards (DBS), concerning such substrates. As such, it is a synthesis of information previously presented by many others and, also, of data derived from studies performed by others under contract funds from DBS. It is hoped in this way to make you aware of the practicalities that face a regulatory agency in the decision-making processes.

The licensing of the poliomyelitis, so-called Salk Vaccine, by the United States in 1955, signaled the start of modern day vaccination against viral diseases. That vaccine was produced from cell cultures prepared from the kidneys of rhesus or cynomolgus monkeys which were caged in groups of 50 to 100, both during transport to the United States and for a varying period of time in manufacturing establishments of biological products prior to removal of kidneys. Such caging facilities provided an ideal situation for the spread of agents from animal to animal. During the 1950's, many viral agents were isolated and studied by Hull *et al* (1-3). As the result of these studies and many others (4,5), it gradually became clear that isolation and quarantine might lead to less contamination of animals with extraneous agents. Thus when regulations were adopted in the United States for Poliovirus Vaccine, Live, Oral (Sabin Vaccine) (6) requirements were established for a rigorous six-week period of quarantine and conditioning of the animals used to provide the vaccine substrate. Nevertheless, while the situation improved, some extraneous agents could still be found and it is now clear that agents such as foamy virus, SV-40 and simian cytomegalovirus are indigenous to rhesus, cynomolgus, and African green monkeys (4,5,7) much as many viruses are indigenous in man (8,9). Of prime importance, of course, is the effect of such indigenous agents in terms of the cell substrates which are used for the production of viral vaccines. Regulations (6) for poliovirus vaccine require elaborate and intensive testing both of the cell culture systems and the virus pools for the presence of such extraneous agents. Nevertheless, prior to 1960, vaccines which were produced in rhesus monkey kidney cell cultures were subsequently found to contain an agent which was not known at that time. This virus was described by Sweet and Hilleman in 1960 (7) and was later identified as the oncogenic substance (10) first described by Eddy *et al* (11) which caused sarcomas in newborn hamsters. Since SV-40, furthermore, can cause transformation *in vitro* of cells of many species, including human, (12-15) and since it was demonstrated to be present in inactivated poliomyelitis vaccine (16), new regulations were quickly adopted to specifically exclude SV-40 from all vaccines subsequently produced in monkey kidney cell cultures.

But, what of the individuals who had received the vaccines so contaminated? What studies could be done to indicate the outcome of receiving such materials? With the information available, only retrospective epidemiologic studies were possible. In this regard, the results of the study reported in 1963 by Fraumeni *et al* (17) indicated no difference in mortality rates due to malignancies between children receiving contaminated poliomyelitis vaccine and those receiving poliomyelitis vaccine free of SV-40. Even more recently, Fraumeni and his colleagues (18) reported data on an eight-year follow-up of 787 newborn infants most of whom received Poliovirus Vaccine, Live, Oral, less than three days after birth. In addition, there was a small group of 137 newborns who received Inactivated Poliomyelitis Vaccine intramuscularly. This vaccine also contained a substantial quantity of SV-40. In this group of 918 children, eight years later, there were no deaths from cancer although the expected value was 0.6 computed by a modified life-table analysis based on published death rates in the area where the study was performed.

Such retrospective studies are, of course, less satisfactory than prospective studies would be. However, at present, no other methodology can be used to follow persons involved in past clinical trials. The information obtained, while not absolutely conclusive, certainly indicates that, at present, there is no evidence that SV-40 is oncogenic for humans even when given to newborn infants.

Other retrospective studies have also yielded valuable information concerning the long range effect of biological products. For example, based on animal studies cited above, one might postulate that the newborn infant would be highly susceptible to the action of a human oncogenic virus. Such an agent might, indeed, be present in the blood and tissues of many healthy individuals in much the same way that the animal leukemia viruses are (19). If the blood of such infected individuals were transfused into highly susceptible newborns, the stage would be set for the possible future development of neoplasms. Therefore, retrospective studies of groups of children who had received exchange transfusions because of *Erythroblastosis fetalis* were initiated and the data obtained were compared with those for control groups matched by sex, race, birth weight, and order of birth in the family. Since the latent period for the development of neoplasia may be very long, follow-up was carried out on persons who had received such therapy during the previous twenty years. Two such studies, performed under contracts from DBS, one in Pittsburgh, Pennsylvania, and one in Minneapolis, Minnesota were undertaken. These studies were more successful than might have been anticipated, in that follow-up was better than 80 percent in both the study and control groups. Among the 3,496 children who had had exchange transfusions as newborns, there were four who had died of acute leukemia. Among four thousand children in the control group, only two had died of acute leukemia. No other significant neoplasms were noted. These studies are inconclusive, since the number of children studied was small; however, it is clear that there was no great increase in leukemia in those children who had received the exchange transfusions.

Another retrospective study has been undertaken in order to assess the long-range effects of Measles Virus Vaccine, Live, Attenuated as used in the field trials done with this product in the State of Maryland between 1959 and 1963. Live Measles Vaccine, as licensed in the United States, is produced using either of two cell substrates, chick embryo or canine renal cells. In 1963, when Live Measles Vaccine was licensed, the need for quarantine of animals was clear. Thus regulations (20) adopted for this product specified the following:

Chick embryo cell cultures:

"Embryonated chicken eggs used as the source of chick embryo tissue for the propagation of measles virus shall be derived from flocks certified to be free of Salmonella pulorum, avian tuberculosis, fowl pox, Rous sarcoma, avian leucosis and other adventitious agents pathogenic for chickens."

Canine renal cell cultures:

"Only dogs in overt good health which have been maintained in quarantine in vermin-proof quarters for a minimum of six months, having had no exposure to other dogs or animals throughout the quarantine period, or dogs born to dogs while so quarantined, provided the progeny have been kept in the same type of quarantine continuously from birth, shall be used as a source of kidney tissue for the propagation of measles virus."

Dogs used for experimental purposes:

"Dogs that have been used previously for experimental or testing purposes with microbiological agents shall not be used as a source of kidney tissue in the manufacture of vaccine. Each dog shall be examined periodically during the quarantine period as well as at the time of necropsy under the direction of a qualified pathologist, physician or veterinarian having experience with diseases of dogs, for the presence of signs or symptoms of ill health, particularly for evidence of tuberculosis, infectious canine hepatitis, canine distemper, rabies, leptospirosis, and other diseases indigenous to dogs. If there are any such signs, symptoms, or other significant pathological lesions observed, tissue from such animals shall not be used in the manufacture of Measles Virus Vaccine, Live, Attenuated."

Although the quarantine procedures for animals such as chickens and dogs are certainly more stringent than those which can be instituted for monkeys, there was still concern that vaccine produced on such cell substrates could induce neoplasms in the children to whom it was administered. Thus, 7,132 children were surveyed during 1968 and 1969, five to ten years after administration of vaccine. Of these, 4,000 received measles vaccine propagated in canine renal cell cultures and 3,132 measles vaccine derived from chick embryo cell culture. The strain of virus and the passage level were identical. The largest number of children were between two and six years of age when the vaccine was administered and 10 and 14 years of age at the time of the surveillance. Only two children with malignant neoplasms were found in this study, both having brain tumors, one an astrocytoma and the other, a medullablastoma. Both had received vaccine prepared in canine renal cells. No leukemic children were found. Although both tumors found were in the brain, the fact that they were of different origin and that the very low frequency is in keeping with expected incidence levels, indicates no evidence for involvement of the vaccine. Further, in these studies, there was no evidence among vaccinated children of subacute sclerosing panencephalitis, a disease related to natural measles infection. Thus, again, the study indicates no significant trends but it cannot be considered completely conclusive.

Although each of these retrospective studies is not completely satisfactory in itself, taken as a group, there is no indication that the use of any of the viral vaccines produced in such varied cell substrates as monkey kidney, canine kidney or chick embryo are causally related to the development of malignant disease.

At present, three new substrates are also being used for the production of viral vaccines; primary duck embryo cell cultures, primary rabbit kidney cell cultures and the human diploid line, WI 38 (21). The use of such a wide variety of cell substrates would appear to be advantageous since prospective comparative follow-up studies could be carried out in the future. Robbins (22) declared, at the Conference on Cell Cultures for Virus Vaccine Production held at NIH in 1967, "I suggest that, in determining what vaccines we will release we attempt to utilize more than one cell source so that we have something to compare to something .... If we vaccinate the total population of children with a vaccine produced in one cell, we do not have a very good base line. If we utilize several different cells or lots of cells, then perhaps we will be able to make some kinds of comparison, assuming we can keep appropriate records." Many others, such as Fox and Murray, agree with this concept (23,24).

As a result of the thoughts expressed above and in order to overcome the disadvantages of retrospective studies, regulations (25) for the newly licensed viral vaccines require that the field studies be performed in a manner that will allow future prospective studies to be carried out.

Thus: "The field studies shall be so conducted that at least 5,000 of the susceptible individuals must reside when inoculated in areas where health related statistics are regularly compiled in accordance with procedures such as those used by the National Center for Health Statistics. Data in such form as will identify each inoculated person shall be furnished to the Director, Division of Biologics Standards."

The data that are to be supplied include the name of the vaccine, age, sex, race, identifying number (such as the Social Security Number in the United States), parents' names including mother's unmarried name and address at time of vaccination. At any time in the future, using data linkage systems, prospective studies can be performed. Dr. Robert Miller, an epidemiologist in the National Cancer Institute, has been attempting to establish in the United States a National Death Index, consisting of a list of all deaths occurring each year arranged alphabetically (26). One could match the data obtained concerning vaccinees with this list and hopefully obtain useful information. While as yet there is no such listing, or what would be even more useful, an index of various types of morbidity, it is hoped that, by collecting the appropriate data now, when studies of current vaccines are done in five to ten years' time such record linkage systems will be available.

In terms of decision-making in the approval of vaccines produced in certain cell culture systems, the retrospective studies have certainly been of importance. For instance, in 1969, at the International Conference on Rubella Immunization held at NIH, Sabin (27) expressed concern "that human embryonic fibroblast cultures" (such as WI 38 cells) "would be the very ones to contain" a human leukemia agent. While there is still no specific evidence to invalidate this supposition, the retrospective studies on the safety of human tissues and blood, as exemplified in the exchange transfusion studies, gave confidence that WI 38 cells could be used for vaccine production. So, after long and careful consideration, approval was given on the first of March for the use of a Poliovirus Vaccine, Live, Oral, produced on human diploid cells in the United States. The clinical trials for this vaccine were also performed in such a way that prospective follow-up studies can be done in the future.

Furthermore, one of the conclusions of the Conference on Cell Cultures for Virus Vaccine Production held at NIH in 1967 was expressed by the Conference Chairman, Dr. Donald Merchant as follows: "It is the sense of the majority of those attending the Conference that we recognize the value of cell lines that can be obtained from selected tissues, that can be carefully controlled, that can be exhaustively studied and tested and that retain normal characteristics. ....A number of lines similar to WI 38 should be developed from human, nonhuman primate and other animal sources so that, as more information is obtained and the need for a wider variety of vaccines is apparent, we will have an ample number and variety of systems with which to work. A number of participants pointed out that we should not have all our eggs in one basket." (28).

With this as a mandate, the Division of Biologics Standards undertook attempts to develop such cell lines, as contracted research projects. Based on our knowledge of what cells might be most useful, two broad areas have been investigated. The development of a rabbit diploid cell line is still in its early stages and there is no data to present as yet. The other, started in 1969, is the development of nonhuman primate diploid cell lines. This work has been performed by Miss Rosalyn Wallace and Dr. Paul Vasington of Lederle Laboratories under the supervision of, and with the cooperation and help of, Doctors John Petricciani and Douglas Lorenz and Mrs. Hope Hopps of DBS. Since a paper describing this work was presented at the International Congress for Microbiological Standardization in Annecy, France (29) and there have been several other publications (30,31), I shall only summarize the work thus far in order to bring the program into focus in relationship to previous remarks and to put it into perspective as far as the Division is concerned.

Since the Division undertook this program as a mandate from the scientific community, based on the conclusions of the cell culture conference of 1967, the developmental program, although performed under contract, is inherently an extension of the programs of DBS. As work has progressed, several nonhuman primate lines have seemed promising and, in order to gain wider experience with these cells, the Division made them available to any interested investigators in December, 1970. It should be pointed out that, in order to assure their availability to all members of the scientific community and interested manufacturing establishments, these cells are the property of the United States Government and are distributed only by DBS.

Now as to some information concerning them: Priority was given to the development of cell lines from Rhesus (*Macaca mulatta*) and African green (*Cercopithecus aethiops*) monkeys. Fetuses were obtained by Caesarian section from carefully screened, quarantined, monkeys of both species. The animals chosen were found to be free of antibody to most viruses such as SV-40, polioviruses, and measles but had low levels of antibody to simian cytomegalovirus and foamy virus. Screening of a large number of animals indicated that it would be impossible to obtain monkeys with no evidence of such antibody.

Although cultures of a number of organs were established only those from lung tissue developed into cell lines which appeared promising. Originally two lines, one from a rhesus and one from an African green, appeared to have the desired characteristics as regards growth potential, susceptibility to viruses, suitability for virus growth, and cytogenetic characteristics. Recently, after study by several investigators, it became evident that the line from the African green monkey, the DBS-FCL-1, becomes quite aneuploid at passage 30. Although this high level of aneuploidy drops from 50 percent at this passage level to 12-18 percent by passages 34-36, it is no longer considered a promising candidate and I shall confine the rest of my remarks to the rhesus monkey diploid line DBS-FRhL-2. Table 1 summarizes the characteristics of this line as of September, 1971. Extensive studies, using methods involving inoculation of many primary and continuous lines with supernatant fluids and cells, inoculation of a variety of laboratory animals, electron microscopic examination of thin sections, and fluorescent antibody techniques, have not revealed the presence of any adventitious agents in FRhL-2.

At present, this cell line has been distributed to 44 laboratories, many have written to us concerning their evaluations of it, and we hope to obtain further information soon. It is gratifying that only three of the large number of laboratories reporting back have had difficulty with the cells. It is too early to

TABLE I

BIOLOGICAL CHARACTERISTICS OF SELECTED CELL LINE DBS-FRhL-2

Tissue	Fetal lung, male rhesus (*Macaca mulatta*).
Passage History	Finite life span to 50 passages. Split ratio 1:3 at passages 1-44; 1:2 at 45-50.
Cell Morphology	Fibroblastic.
Cytogenetics	2N = 42; diploid through passage 36. Polyploidy varying from 0.3 - 1.3%. (Independent of passage level).
Virus Growth	Sensitive: (virus titers similar to that seen in control cultures). Poliovirus 1, 2, 3, Coxsackie A9, parainfluenza 3, rubella, mumps, vaccinia, rhinovirus HGP. Refractory: (Virus titers less than obtained in control cultures). Adenovirus 3, 4, 7, parainfluenza 1 and 2, influenza A2, herpes simplex, measles, CMV, rabies.

determine the final use of such material; the project is continuing in order to gain further data on DBS-FRhL-2 and also to develop an African green line in our attempt to answer the needs outlined above.

SUMMARY

The chronological development of studies concerning viral vaccines and production cell substrates, as viewed from the vantage of hindsight, has been presented. It is clear that such a view is not the most preferable one, and that, presently, with the fore-sight gained by experience future vaccination programs can be planned.

REFERENCES

1. HULL, R.N., MINNER, J.R. & SMITH, J.W. *Am. J. Hyg.* *63*:204, 1956.
2. HULL, R.N. & MINNER, J.R. *Ann. N.Y. Acad. Sci.* *67*:413, 1957.
3. HULL, R.N., MINNER, J.R. & MASCOLI, C.C. *Am. J. Hyg.* *68*: 31, 1958.
4. RUSTIGIAN, R., JOHNSTON, P. & REIHART, H. *Proc. Soc. Exper. Biol. Med.* *88*:8, 1955.
5. MALHERBE, H. & HARWIN, R. *Brit. J. Exper. Path.* *38*:539, 1957.
6. U.S. Department of Health, Education and Welfare, United States Public Health Service Regulations for the Manufacture of Biological Products, Title 42, Part 73, revised 1961.
7. SWEET, B.H. & HILLEMAN, M.R. *Proc. Soc. Exper. Biol. Med.* *105*:420, 1960.
8. ROWE, W.P., HARTLEY, J.W., CRAMBLETT, H.G. & MASTROTA, F.M. *Am. J. Hyg.* *67*:57, 1958.
9. ASHKENASCZI, A. & MELNICK, J.L. *Am. J. Clin. Path.* *38*:209, 1962.
10. EDDY, B.E., BORMAN, G.S., GRUBBS, G. & YOUNG, R.D. *Virology* *17*:65, 1962.
11. EDDY, B.E., BORMAN, G.S., BERKELEY, W. & YOUNG, R.D. *Proc. Soc. Exper. Biol. Med.* *107*:191, 1961.
12. KOPROWSKI, H., PONTÉN, J.A., JENSEN, F., RAVDIN, R.G., MOORHEAD, P. & SAKSELA, E. *J. Cell. Comp. Physiol.* *59*: 281, 1962.
13. RABSON, A.S. & KIRSCHSTEIN, R.L. *Proc. Soc. Exper. Biol. Med.* *111*:323, 1962.
14. SHEIN, H.M. & ENDERS, J.F. *Proc. Nat. Acad. Sci.* *48*:1164, 1962.
15. BLACK, P.H. *Virology* *28*:760, 1966.
16. GERBER, P., HOTTLE, G.A. & GRUBBS, R.E. *Proc. Soc. Exper. Biol. Med.* *108*:205, 1961.
17. FRAUMENI, J.F., EDERER, F. & MILLER, R.W. *J.A.M.A.* *185*: 713, 1963.
18. FRAUMENI, J.F., STARK, C.R., GOLD, E. & LEPOW, M.L. *Science* *167*:59, 1970.
19. KAPLAN, H.S. *Nat. Cancer Inst. Mono.* *4*:141, 1960.
20. U.S. Department of Health, Education and Welfare, United States Public Health Service Regulations for the Manufacture of Biological Products, Title 42, Part 73, revised 1963.
21. HAYFLICK, L. & MOORHEAD, P.S. *Exper. Cell Res.* *25*:585, 1961.
22. ROBBINS, F.C. *Nat. Cancer Inst. Mono.* *29*:457, 1968.
23. FOX, J.P. *Nat. Cancer Inst. Mono.* *29*:459, 1968.
24. MURRAY, R. *Nat. Cancer Inst. Mono.* *29*:460, 1968.
25. U.S. Department of Health, Education and Welfare, United States Public Health Service Regulations for the Manufacture of Biological Products, Title 42, Part 73, revised 1969.

26. MILLER, R.W. *Nat. Cancer Inst. Mono.* *29*:453, 1968.
27. SABIN, A.B. Discussion, Proceedings of the International Conference on Rubella Immunization, p. 378. National Institute of Health, Bethesda, Md., Feb. 18-20, 1969.
28. MERCHANT, D.J. *Nat. Cancer Inst. Mono.* *29*:583, 1968.
29. WALLACE, R.E., VASINGTON, P.J. & PETRICCIANI, J.C. Diploid cell lines from sub-human primates as substrates for vaccine production, Twelfth International Congress of the International Association of Microbiological Societies, Permanent Section for Microbiological Standardization, September, 1971, Annecy, France.
30. PETRICCIANI, J.C., HOPPS, H.E. & LORENZ, D.E. *Science* *174*: 1025, 1971.
31. WALLACE, R.E., VASINGTON, P.J., PETRICCIANI, J.C., HOPPS, H.E., & LORENZ, D.E. (To be published.)

VACCINATION WITH PURIFIED VIRAL PROTEINS

H. G. Pereira

Division of Virology, National Institute for Medical Research, Mill Hill
London, England

Inactivated viral vaccines currently in use consist, in most cases, of rather impure suspensions of virus particles and soluble antigens. It has been demonstrated that not all antigens of a given virus are required to induce antibody responses leading to protection. The useful proteins present in most vaccines represent, therefore, only a small proportion of their total macromolecular composition. This applies even to the best vaccines consisting of purified suspensions of intact or disrupted virus particles. The use of vaccines containing only the purified viral components required for protection will have the following advantages:

1. It will eliminate superfluous proteins which may cause undesirable sensitization or toxic reactions.

2. It will avoid the inoculation of viral nucleic acid which, even if lacking infectivity, might retain undesirable coding potential.

3. It will make possible the use of higher immunizing doses.

4. It will make it possible for vaccine standardization to be based on chemical as well as biological criteria.

Although considerable effort has been directed towards the development of pure viral protein vaccines, no preparation of this type is yet available except at the experimental level. Commercial production may be made possible by the use of virus strains with exceptionally high growth capacity and by the development of improved techniques for the purification of the desired proteins.

SYNTHETIC VACCINES - A DREAM OR REALITY

Ruth Arnon

Department of Chemical Immunology
The Weizmann Institute of Science
Rehovot, Israel

A great deal of information has been presented at this conference concerning vaccination and vaccines. This has included modification and improvement of known vaccine preparations or the route of vaccination; the possible use of virus subunits or purified virus proteins in vaccination; and the development of new vaccines with specificities different than those used hitherto. A great effort is being invested in this field, and indeed many vaccines are being developed; but there are many more viruses which still await an efficient vaccination procedure.

Although vaccines have been highly rewarding in providing immunity, there are several drawbacks to the vaccination methods that are presently used. For example, while in some cases killed vaccines may provide adequate immunity, in others it is essential to use the live attenuated vaccine. But it is not known whether successful live attenuated vaccines can be prepared for a large number of viruses; nor is the reason for these difficulties understood. There is, therefore, no way of predicting the conditions for preparation of any particular vaccine. In addition, one cannot overlook the hazard of infection that is involved in the use of live vaccines and the rigorous measures for quality control that are, therefore, required during the process of their production. Another major disadvantage in contemporary vaccine use is the narrow specificity of the protection afforded, which is limited to the particular virus used in the vaccine. Thus, each strain of virus requires a separate vaccine. Considering the recent steady increase in expression of new virus strains having differing specificities, there is a persistent increase in the number of vaccines that have to be developed. Clearly, to cope with the problem of the overwhelming number of vaccines which will be needed in the future, fundamentally new approaches to vaccination are required. This problem may not seem urgent today, but it will be unavoidable and inescapable in ten or twenty years, and an early start towards exploring other approaches is indicated.

In this paper I would like to suggest a possible approach - namely, the use of synthetic macromolecules as multivalent vaccines. It should be emphasized that if it turns out that the use of live attenuated vaccines is a universal solution for all cases of viral diseases, the whole synthetic approach will be superfluous. However, if killed vaccines continue to be an important vehicle for immunization, the following approach should be of interest. I would like to start by describing the scientific background and experimental data on which we base our hopes that such an approach is feasible, and subsequently to outline the anticipated advantages and possible drawbacks it might encompass.

Before attempting to synthesize a vaccine we should be clear about the exact criteria of its evaluation. Vaccination, in general, involves the use of an immunizing agent, which is expected to elicit protection, namely, the formation of neutralizing antibodies against a biologically active material such as a bacterium, virus, or toxin. The immunizing agent comprises usually the intact organism, in a killed or attenuated form. The mechanism of this protection is not known, neither is it known whether all the antibodies elicited by the vaccine participate in the neutralization process. Moreover, these questions are not easily amenable to experimental elucidation due to the huge size and complexity of the immunizing agent molecule. It seems, thus, that we are almost in the dark concerning the most basic phenomenon involved in the vaccination process - neutralization.

In order to shed some light on the problem of neutralization of biologically active molecules by their specific antibodies, recourse has been made to model systems using as antigens simpler molecules possessing biological activity. Enzymes seem to be suitable for such a purpose, for the following reasons: They can be readily isolated in a pure state and their structure can be elucidated; indeed, both the primary and the three dimensional structure of several enzymes have been established (1-3); accurate sensitive methods are available for assaying their biological, namely, catalytic activity. The mode of action of many enzymes has also been elucidated, as well as the composition and structure of their active sites (e.g., lysozyme (4)). Hence, the mechanism of their neutralization by antibodies may be interpreted on a molecular level.

Principally, neutralization can occur via three mechanisms: (a) a direct interaction of the antibodies with the active site; (b) interaction of the antibodies with regions contiguous or adjacent to the active site, i.e., steric hindrance; and (c) by interaction with other regions, in a manner which either induces conformational changes in the molecule, leading to loss of catalytic activity, or prevents conformational changes induced by the substrate to allow the active conformation of the catalytic site. Studies with many different enzyme systems have indicated that the prevailing mechanism is steric hindrance (5). This has been demonstrated both by kinetic studies illustrating the pure non-competitive characteristics of the enzyme inactivation by antibodies (6), and by the finding that in most enzyme-anti-enzyme systems there is a correlation between the size of the substrate and the extent of inactivation (5) as illustrated for the system trypsin - antitrypsin in Fig. 1. However, there is no unified concept for the mechanism of inhibition of all enzymes, and, depending on the particular system studied, the two other mechanisms may be manifested as well.

An important feature characterizing the inhibition of enzymes by their respective antibodies is the residual catalytic activity persisting even when there is a great excess of antibody, and which is not reduced by the addition of more antibody. This phenomenon is also depicted in Fig. 1, especially for the low molecular weight substrate. These findings can be interpreted in at least two ways. One possible explanation is that each enzyme molecule is partially inhibited by the antibody, while retaining some residual activity. Alternatively, the antibody population could be considered as being inherently heterogeneous, consisting of species which differ in their inhibitory capacity. The validity of this second premise was demonstrated in studies with several enzyme systems by the separation of the antibodies to fractions that differed in their inhibitory capacities (7,8).

In our studies on anti-papain antibodies (9,10), we achieved such fractionation on the basis of the capability of the antibodies to cross-react with a related enzyme, chymopapain, which contains similar antigenic determinants. The two related enzymes, papain and chymopapain, in this case show 10-20 percent cross reaction in the precipitin reaction, and are also cross-inactivated by their respective antisera. It could, therefore, be assumed that the common regions in their molecules include those antigenic determinants whose interaction with the antibodies is responsible for the decrease in catalytic activity. Indeed, fractionation of anti-papain antibodies by cross-adsorption on chymopapain immunoadsorbent yielded a fraction which possessed an inhibitory capacity much greater than that of the total purified antibody preparation. On the other hand, the antibodies that could not bind to chymopapain and were subsequently isolated on papain immunoadsorbent, although

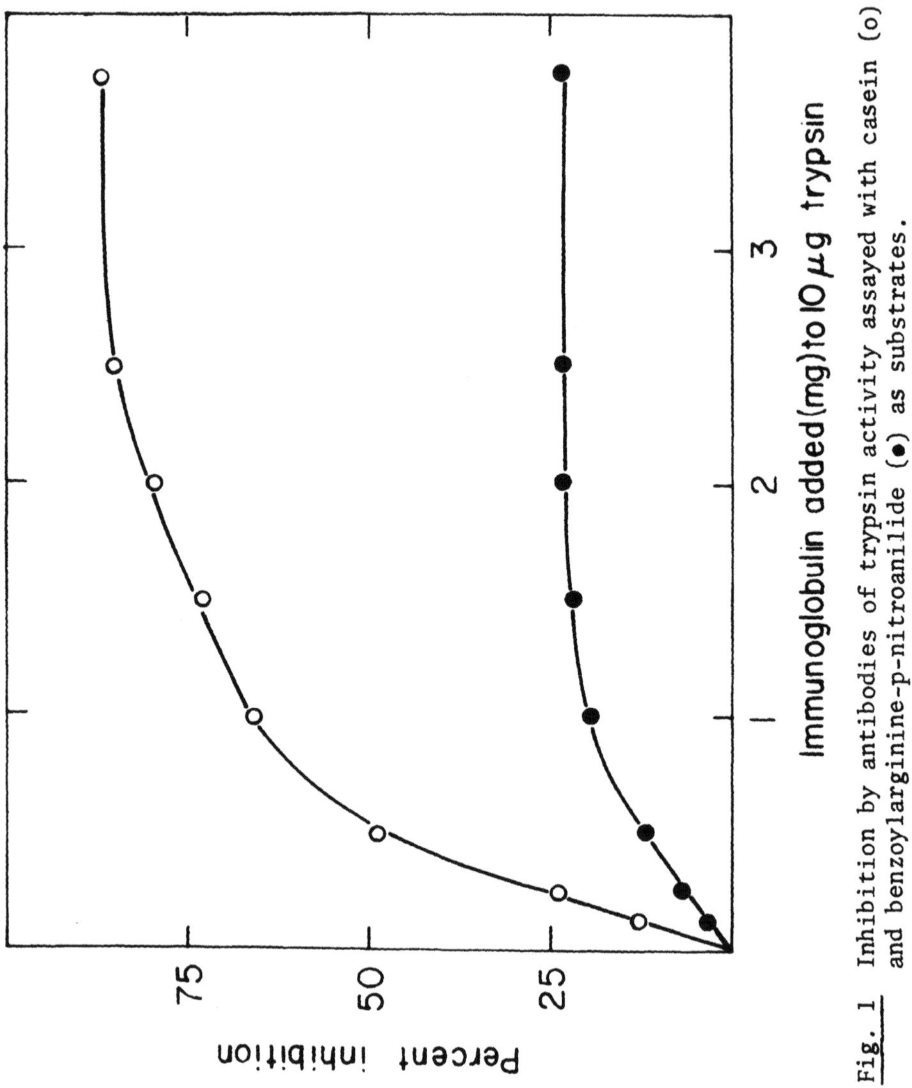

Fig. 1 Inhibition by antibodies of trypsin activity assayed with casein (o), and benzoylarginine-p-nitroanilide (●) as substrates.

excellent precipitating antibodies, were hardly inhibitory at all (Fig. 2).

An experiment of this kind mainly demonstrates that even with a relatively low molecular weight, and simple, biologically active material such as papain, only 10-20 percent of the antibodies are neutralizing, the remainder being inert as far as neutralization is concerned. The same phenomenon should certainly also exist in the case of toxins and viruses, and might prove of practical value in the preparation of antisera for passive anti-toxin immunization.

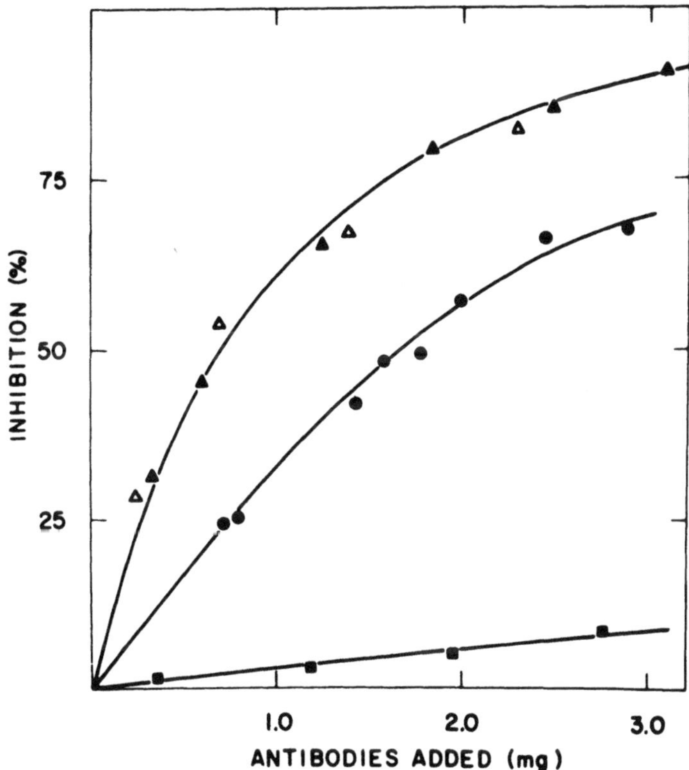

Fig. 2 Inhibition of the enzymatic activity of papain (50 μg) on benzoyl-L-arginine ethyl ester by the total anti-papain antibodies preparation (●) and by the two selectively fractionated species, i.e., the fraction that was isolated on chymopapain immunoadsorbent (▲), and the antibodies that could not bind to chymopapain immunoadsorbent (■). The open triangles (Δ) indicate the inhibition of chymopapain (50 μg) by the fraction of anti-papain antibodies that was isolated on chymopapain immunoadsorbent.

It is known that some toxins, such as snake venoms of different species, display immunological cross-reaction. It is reasonable to assume that the regions shared by such cross-reacting toxins - when they possess similar toxic properties - might be related to their toxic activity. If the cross-reaction were used for fractionation of antibodies from the antisera, it is possible that the common fraction would be of much higher anti-toxin capacity and might be more efficacious in therapeutic use.

The fact that only a small percentage of the antibodies participates in neutralization has another very important implication; if we were able to find means whereby to elicit only the neutralizing antibodies, we would get much more efficient protective immunization.

The first step towards this goal was to determine whether it is feasible to elicit antibodies specific towards a unique limited region in a macromolecule. We have carried out studies in this direction recently in collaboration with Prof. Michael Sela, on hen egg-white lysozyme. Lysozyme is particularly suitable for immunological studies due to the detailed information available on its primary as well as its spatial structure, and the comprehension of its mode of action (4). By a combination of limited proteolysis and mild reduction, an immunologically active fragment of the molecule was isolated (11). This fragment, consisting of residues 60-83 in the amino acid sequence of lysozyme (Fig. 3) and containing one intrachain disulfide bond, was denoted "loop". Antibodies specific to this region only were selectively isolated from anti-lysozyme serum by adsorption on an appropriate "loop" immunoadsorbent. The anti-"loop" antibodies thus isolated showed, as expected, less heterogeneity than the total anti-lysozyme antibodies.

Antibodies with the same specificity could be prepared by an alternative, more interesting procedure. The isolated "loop" peptide was attached to a synthetic macromolecular carrier (multichain poly-DL-alanine) and the resultant semi-synthetic conjugates served for immunization of rabbits and goats. The antibodies elicited were reactive with lysozyme and thus purified anti-"loop" antibodies were isolated from this antiserum by adsorption on lysozyme. More detailed specificity studies demonstrated that these antibodies were directed towards a conformation-dependent determinant. This was indicated both by their ability to recognize the "loop" structure in native lysozyme, and by their capability of distinguishing between the "loop" and its open peptide chain. These findings were established using three different techniques (12): antigen-binding experiments, inactivation of modified bacteriophage, and the inhibition of excitation energy transfer from the anti-"loop" antibodies to a "loop" derivative to which dimethyl aminonaphthalene-5-sulfonyl (dansyl) groups were attached (13). The results obtained by this

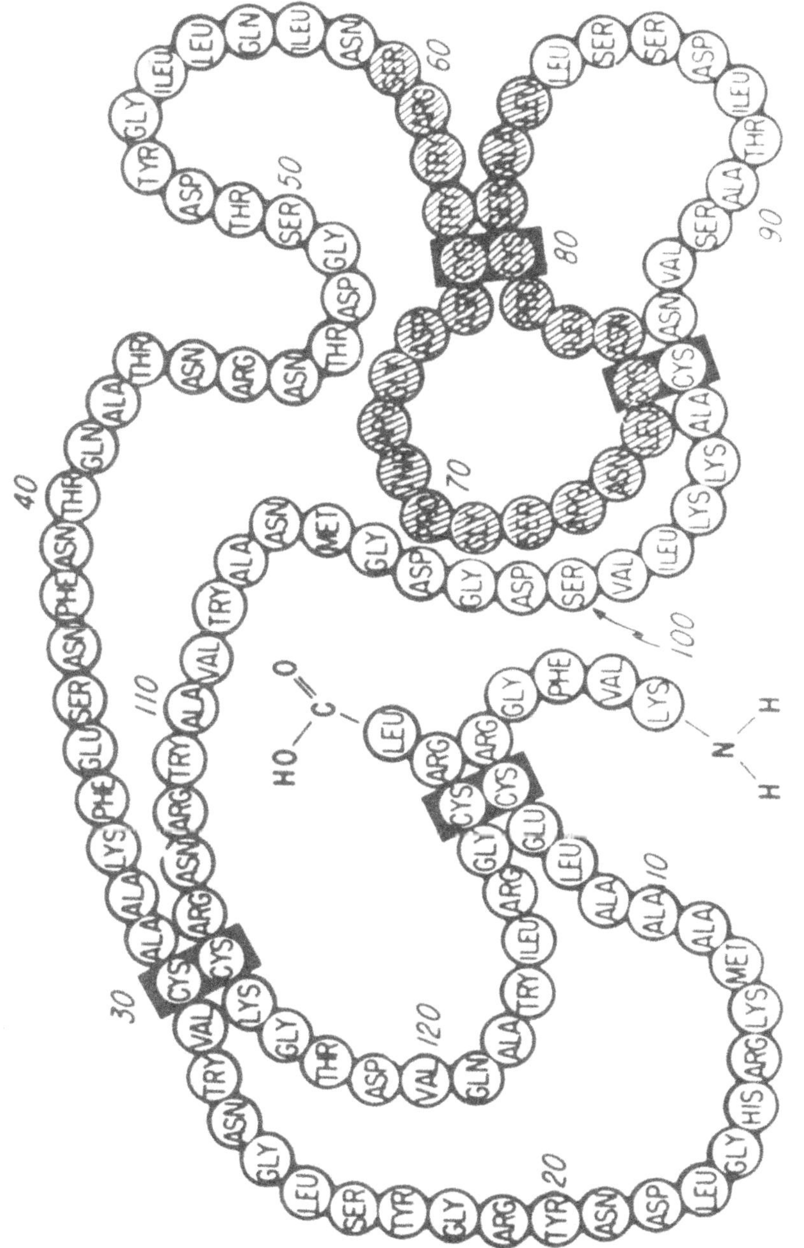

Fig. 3 Amino acid sequence of hen egg-white lysozyme. The region of the "loop" peptide is shaded.

last-mentioned technique, using fluorescence measurements, were as follows: The specific interaction between the antibodies and the dansyl-"loop" derivative was manifested by enhancement of the fluorescence. As seen in Fig. 4, the "loop" peptide was capable of inhibiting this enhancement, as was intact lysozyme, which was as effective as the "loop" on a molar basis. The open peptide chain of the "loop", in which the disulfide bond was disrupted by reduction and alkylation, was not reactive at all. From this and additional evidence it is, therefore, clear that the anti-"loop" antibodies interact with native lysozyme via the "loop" structure in it.

Since the amino acid sequence of the "loop" region is completely established, it was of interest to check whether a similar peptide, prepared synthetically, would have the same action. The chemical synthesis of a "loop"-like peptide (14) was carried out in collaboration with Prof. C. B. Anfinsen of the National Institutes of Health, Bethesda, Md., U.S.A., according to Merrifield's procedure (15), as illustrated in Fig. 5. A conjugate was subsequently prepared by attaching the resultant "loop" peptide to the synthetic carrier, namely, multichain poly-DL-alanine. Immunization with this conjugate yielded antibodies similar in every respect to those elicited by the conjugate of the natural lysozyme "loop", as illustrated in Fig. 6, using again inhibition of fluorescence enhancement as the measuring technique.

We have thus shown that, at least in the case of lysozyme, it is possible to use a completely synthetic molecule for eliciting antibodies reactive with a native protein; moreover, these antibodies are directed toward a unique, conformation-dependent, limited region in the protein. Regretably, in this case the anti-"loop" antibodies did not possess anti-catalytic activity. It should be possible, however, in similar studies to use fragments that will elicit inhibitory antibodies.

If this is possible for one enzyme, there is no theoretical reason why similar results cannot be obtained with any other enzyme of which the amino acid sequence is known, such as for example, bacteriophage lysozyme. One might predict that it may be possible to prepare synthetic molecules that will provoke an immune response against the bacteriophage enzyme, and thus produce anti-viral antibody. Clearly, the next step is to approach in a similar manner other more complicated viruses which are of more direct interest to man, for example, the neuraminidase of influenza virus described in this Symposium by Dr. Laver. The approach is of course not limited to molecules with enzymatic activity: it can apply also to any other viral coat protein which participates in the immunological activity of the virus.

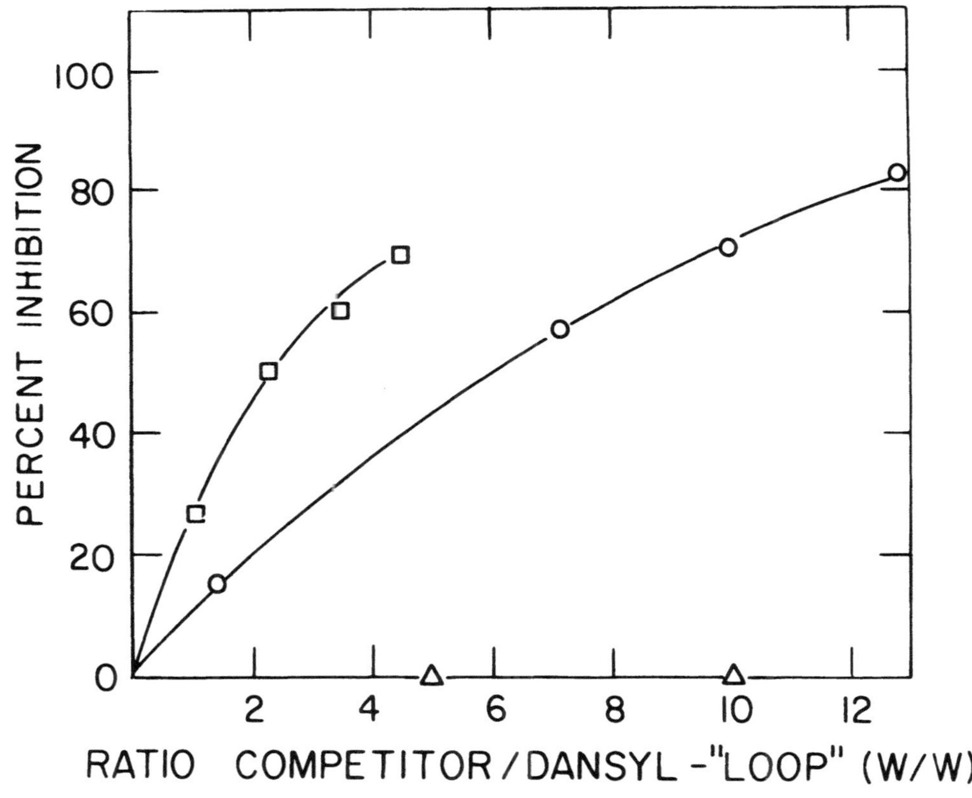

Fig. 4 Inhibition of the enhanced fluorescence of the mixture of dansyl "loop" (4 μM) and anti-"loop" antibodies (0.6 μM), by varying concentrations of the "loop" peptide (□) hen egg-white lysozyme (o), and the open-chain peptide obtained by reduction and carboxymethylation of the "loop" peptide (Δ).

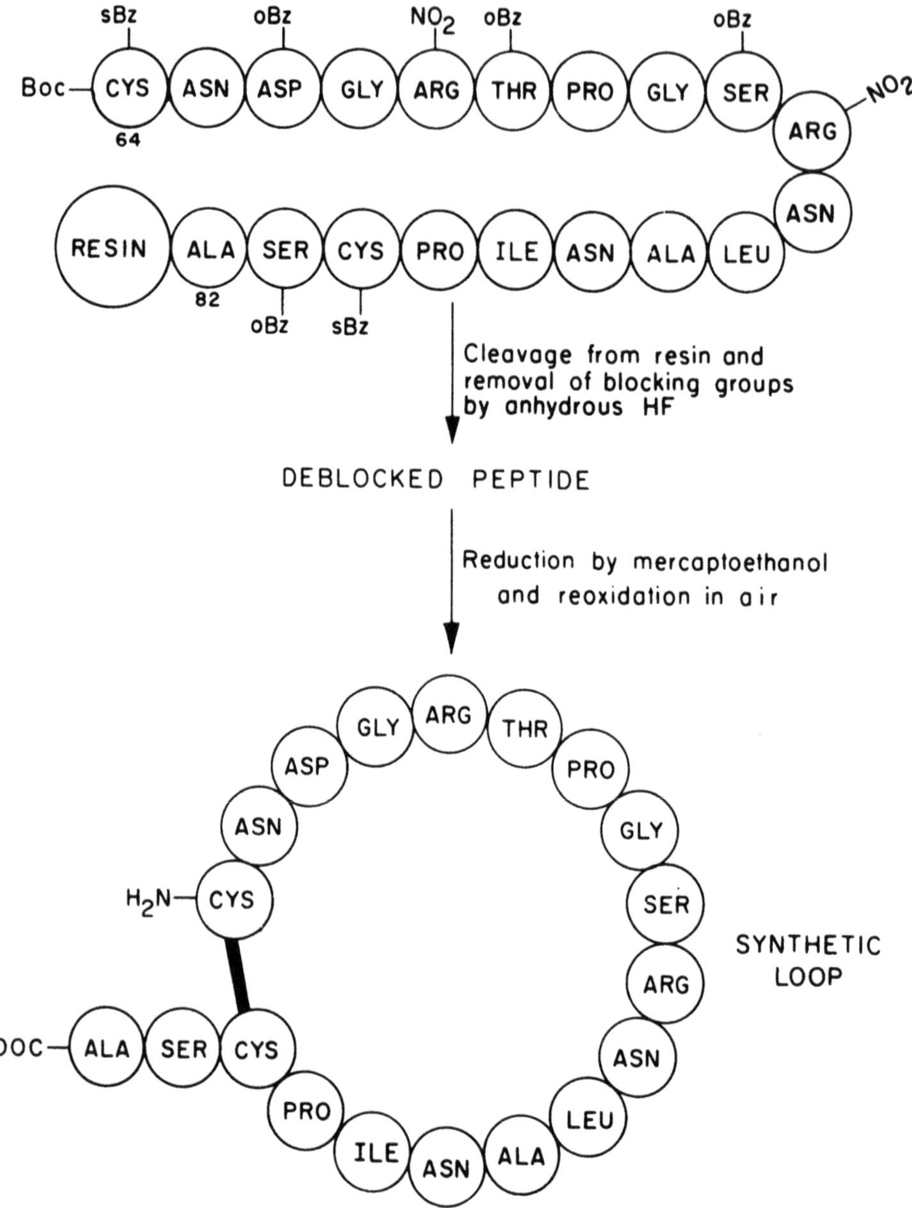

Fig. 5 Scheme of solid-phase synthesis of the "loop" peptide of lysozyme, consisting of residues 64-82. Cys-76 was replaced by alanine; Gly-67 was radioactively labeled.

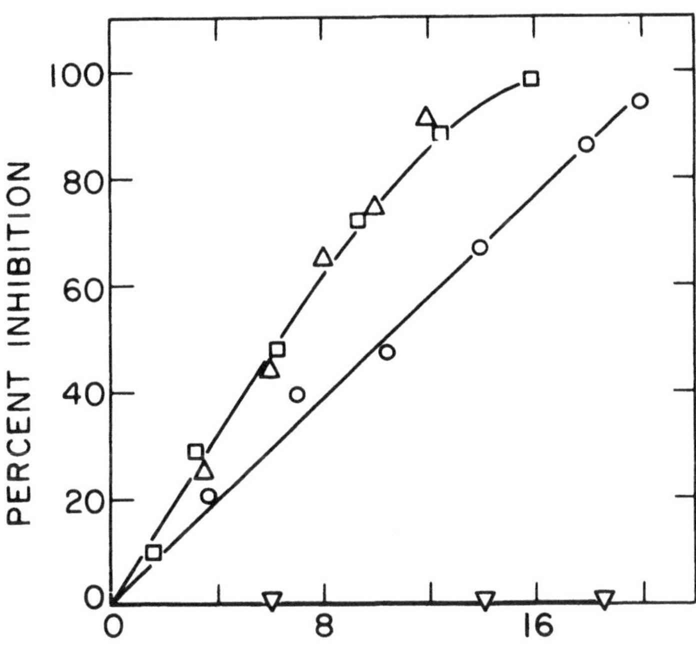

Fig. 6 Inhibition of the enhanced fluorescence of a mixture of dansyl-"loop" (2.5 μM) and antisynthetic "loop" antibodies (0.4 μM), by lysozyme (o), natural "loop" (Δ), synthetic "loop" (□), or performic acid-oxidized synthetic "loop" (∇). The extent of inhibition was calculated from the decrease in the fluorescence at 520 nm.

There are at least two other recent examples in which synthetic macromolecules were used for protective immunization, and those add to our impression that the synthetic approach to vaccination holds future promise. In one recent case, studied in the laboratory of Prof. Westphal in Freiburg, the synthetic immunogen was a macromolecule containing a sugar component of *Salmonella typhi*, O-acetylabequose; it was found capable of provoking antibodies that agglutinate certain strains of *Salmonella*. Studies of the effect of such an antigen on infectivity, and of its possible vaccination effectivity, might serve as an important contribution toward reaching the goal of synthetic vaccines. In the second reported case, a synthetic antigen containing the presumed receptor site of wheat-germ agglutinin (a lectin capable of specifically agglutinating tumor cells), conjugated with methylated serum albumin, was found to elicit an immune response in mice, and was capable of cross-reacting with the receptor sites on tumor-cell surfaces (16). Mice immunized against this antigen were able to reject five times as many transplanted myeloma tumor cells as are rejected by otherwise identically treated control mice. This synthetic antigen can act, therefore, as a "chemical vaccine against tumor progression". From these two recent reports it emerges that the synthetic approach to vaccination is not limited to viruses and may be envisaged in other areas, including anti-cancer vaccines.

Of course, we are now just at the beginning of the road. A prerequisite for the success of the approach is the elucidation of the primary and spatial structure of the viral proteins, followed by the identification of the antigenic determinants which are involved in the process of neutralization by the antibodies. Only then would it become feasible to prepare peptides containing such determinants, either from natural materials, or synthetically, and use them for the manufacture of synthetic vaccines. The ultimate objective would be to attach as many as five or even ten different types of determinants, characteristic of various disease-causing viruses, to one synthetic macromolecule and to use it for immunization in such a way that all the determinants would be equally immunopotent, thus serving for simultaneous vaccination against several diseases.

It is obvious that the approach suggested here may have several drawbacks. First, no information is as yet available about the persistence of an antibody response to synthetic immunogens designed according to the lines discussed above. Second, it is not certain whether it will be successful for all viruses. And lastly, the achievement of large scale applicability of vaccines produced by methods based on this approach may take a long time.

There are on the other hand, several advantages to the synthetic approach over the presently used methods of vaccination.

First, as already mentioned, each adequately designed macromolecule will be "multivalent", and thus able to replace many narrowly-specific vaccines of today. Second, it will eliminate immunization against many irrelevant antigenic determinants of the virus, or irrelevant proteins which contaminate the viral preparation in the vaccine. Thus the frequently occurring undesired side-reactions may be avoided. Third, for many vaccines, the addition of an adjuvant is required in order to initiate the immune response. Some of these adjuvants, such as, for example, peanut oil emulsion, may be less damaging than others, but still may induce undesired side-effects. In a synthetic macromolecule this problem of adjuvanticity may find its solution by the introduction of certain groups which enhance antigenicity. Such groups may include fatty acids such as lauric acid, or amino acid residues such as tyrosine, which are known enhancers of immunogenicity (17,18). Thus the synthetic vaccine will contain built-in adjuvanticity and may prove of less hazard and better quality for human use.

Another advantage of the synthetic approach is the possibility of designing the molecule according to will and need. For example, as was indicated in the lecture by Drs. Mozes and Shearer and Prof. Sela at this meeting, the immune response is genetically controlled. Hence, the capacity to respond toward different antigenic determinants, including the "loop" of lysozyme (19), depends to a great extent on the genetic makeup of the immunized animal. There are indications that in many cases this phenomenon may be linked to the histocompatibility antigens of the host (20) and may be dependent on the carrier macromolecule (21) as well as on the antigenic determinants attached to it. It may thus be foreseen that the efficiency of the synthetic vaccine for persons differing in their histocompatibility antigens may depend on the macromolecular carrier used for its preparation. A detailed study of this correlation might enable the selection of the most efficient vaccine to be used according to tissue typing.

By adequate molecular engineering, all the possible variations of vaccines may be designed, enabling us to have on the shelf a series of different multivalent synthetic vaccines to be used according to a preprogrammed key. This certainly sounds today like a dream. The road will be a very long and difficult one. However, with the increasing pace of accumulation of knowledge concerning the structure of proteins, and the knowhow for their synthesis, it may be hoped that if the proper effort will be invested in research on these lines, this dream may become a reality.

REFERENCES

1. KARTHA, G., BELLO, J. & HARKER, D. *Nature 213:*862, 1967.
2. SIGLER, P.B., BLOW, D.M., MATTHEWS, B.W. & HENDERSON, R. *J. Mol. Biol. 35:*143, 1968.
3. LIPSCOMB, W.N., HARTSUCK, J.A., REEKE, G.N., JR., QUINCHO, F. A., BETHGE, P.H., LUDWIG, M.L. ET AL. *Brookhaven Symp. Biol. 21:*24, 1968.
4. PHILLIPS, D.C. *Proc. Nat. Acad. Sci. 57:*484, 1967.
5. CINADER, B. In: Antibodies to Biologically Active Molecules (B. Cinader Ed.) Pergamon Press, Oxford (1967).
6. SHAPIRA, E. & ARNON, R. *Biochemistry 6:*3951, 1967.
7. POLLOCK, M.R. *Immunology 7:*707, 1964.
8. SUZUKI, T., PELICHOVA, H. & CINADER, B. *J. Immunol. 103:*1366, 1969.
9. ARNON, R. & SHAPIRA, E. *Biochemistry 6:*3942, 1967.
10. ARNON, R. & SHAPIRA, E. *Biochemistry 7:*4196, 1968.
11. ARNON, R. & SELA, M. *Proc. Nat. Acad. Sci. 62:*163, 1969.
12. MARON, E., SHIOZAWA, C., ARNON, R. & SELA, M. *Biochemistry 10:*763, 1971.
13. PECHT, I., MARON, E., ARNON, R. & SELA, M. *Europ. J. Biochem. 18:*469, 1971.
14. ARNON, R., MARON, E., SELA, M. & ANFINSEN, C.B. *Proc. Nat. Acad. Sci. 68:*1450, 1971.
15. MERRIFIELD, B.B. *Science 150:*178, 1965.
16. SHIER, W.T. *Proc. Nat. Acad. Sci. 68:*2078, 1971.
17. RÜDE, E., MEYER-DELUIS, M. & GUNDELACH, M.L. *Europ. J. Immunol. 1:*113, 1971.
18. ARNON, R. & SELA, M. *Biochem. J. 75:*103, 1960.
19. MOZES, E., MARON, E., ARNON, R. & SELA, M. *J. Immunol. 106:*862, 1971.
20. McDEVITT, H.O. & BENACERRAF, B. *Advances in Immunol. 11:*31, 1969.
21. SHEARER, G.M., MOZES, E. & SELA, M. *J. Exp. Med. 135:*1972.

POLIOMYELITIS VACCINATION IN TROPICAL COUNTRIES

W. C. Cockburn

World Health Organization

Geneva, Switzerland

It has been demonstrated on a number of occasions in recent years that so far as poliomyelitis is concerned the world is divided sharply into the have-nots and the haves. The highly developed countries, mainly in the temperate climates, are the have-nots and the developing areas are the haves.

Dr. Drozdov and I,(1-3) using data provided to WHO by national health authorities have attempted to depict the changing state of poliomyelitis in the world over the past two decades. It is not necessary to repeat in detail the figures already published. They are summarized in Table 1, where the average annual number of cases in three quinquennia (1951-55, 1961-65 and 1966-70) are shown for groups of countries in different parts of the world. In the first group - U.S.A., Canada, Australia and New Zealand, there has been a spectacular decrease of 780-fold between the first quinquennium and the third. In 23 countries in Europe there has also been a considerable fall in incidence - of about 40-fold; but in 72 countries in Africa, Central and South America and Asia there has either been an increase or at best, only a slight decrease.

Though this table is useful in providing a summary of our findings it obscures the differences in incidence in individual countries. Dömök (4) has shown diagramatically (Fig. 1a and 1b) the increases or decreases in 1961-65 and 1966-69 over 1951-55 in 31 African countries.

Only eight show decreases - the remaining 23 show increases ranging from two-fold to 15-fold or more. The position in much of Central and South America and Asia is only slightly better than

TABLE I

AVERAGE ANNUAL NUMBER OF
CASES OF POLIOMYELITIS REPORTED TO WHO

Area	No. of Countries	1951-55	1961-65	1966-70
N. America, Australia and New Zealand	4	44,378	852	57
Europe	23	28,359	6,665	732
Africa	35	3,660	3,932	4,005*
Central and South America	20	4,639	3,903	3,055
Asia	17	4,718	4,647	3,912

*1966-69

that in Africa.

In terms of completeness of reporting one can have reasonable confidence in the data from the European countries and from North America, Australia and New Zealand. But this is not the case in most countries in other parts of the world.

Chastel (5) reported that the real incidence in two tropical countries known to him - Cambodia (Khmer Republic) and Senegal - was at least 50 percent greater than that given in one of our papers (1) and Perabo (6) made a similar report about cases in the Ivory Coast. Dömök (4) made a special study of this point in Uganda. During the four-year period 1966-69, in that country 101 cases were officially notified but in the same interval specimens from 296 cases of clinically typical poliomyelitis were investigated in the East African Virus Research Institute - which receives most of its material from one hospital alone. It is known that an epidemic occurred between July 1968 and June 1969. According to the records collected from all the hospitals in Uganda, over 980 cases were diagnosed in this epidemic.

Thus the total cases notified in four years was only about 10 percent of the cases diagnosed by clinicians in one epidemic. The recorded decrease for Uganda shown in Fig. 1 is therefore highly misleading. Instead of a fall there was probably a two-fold or greater rise between 1951-55 and 1966-69. No doubt under-reporting occurs to a greater or lesser extent in many other countries and we may conclude that paralytic poliomyelitis is a disease of great public health importance in many warm-climate countries. Though epidemics of the magnitude seen in Europe and North America in the immediate pre-vaccination era are not yet being experienced, outbreaks of over 500 reported cases are no longer unusual and in some countries 2,000 cases or more have been reported in a single year. In 1968, there were 1,000 paralytic cases in one Indian city alone. Also disquieting is the fact that large outbreaks are beginning to occur once again in areas where vaccination programs were instituted with considerable publicity and enthusiasm several years ago but where the enthusiasm has waned and the proportion of susceptible children has again increased.

There are several reasons for the known increasing incidence of the disease in tropical countries; for example, the high rate of population growth, the falling infant mortality rates and the rapidly increasing urbanization. Better reporting may also play some part.

Another possible factor, mentioned by Gear over 20 years ago and more recently by Sabin (7) and Dömök and Balayan (personal communication) is the dispersion (as a result of increased international travel and population movements) of new strains more virulent than "local" strains.

A third factor - one of the most important - is the failure to establish effective regular vaccination programs. As stated in a recent WHO publication (8) - "The inability to maintain an adequate infant immunization program has been the most distressing weakness of most national health services" (in developing countries). There are of course many explanations of the failure to use to good purpose the most potent of weapons for the rapid prevention of many of the communicable diseases, but discussion of them is not relevant to this paper. However, there are countries in the warm-climate regions which are known to have instituted satisfactory poliomyelitis vaccination schemes and it is shown in Table 2 how the incidence of the disease in these countries compares with that in others.

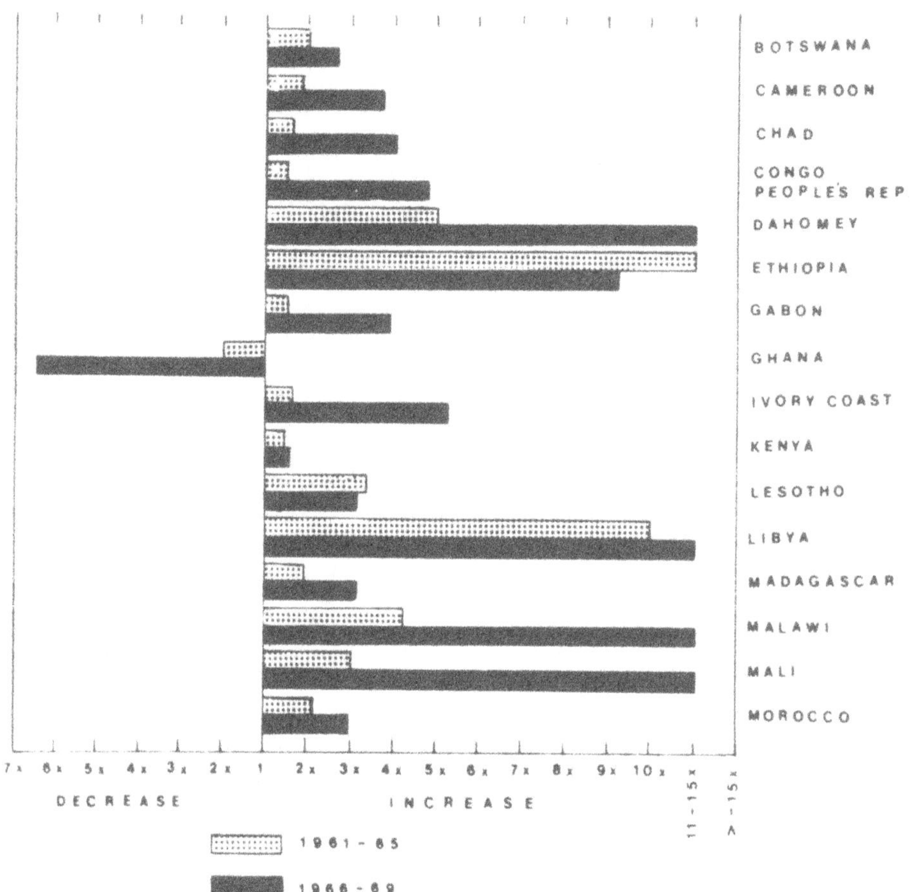

Fig. 1-a Changes in incidence of poliomyelitis in 31 African countries during the periods 1961-65 and 1966-69 as compared to 1951-55. (From Reference 4)

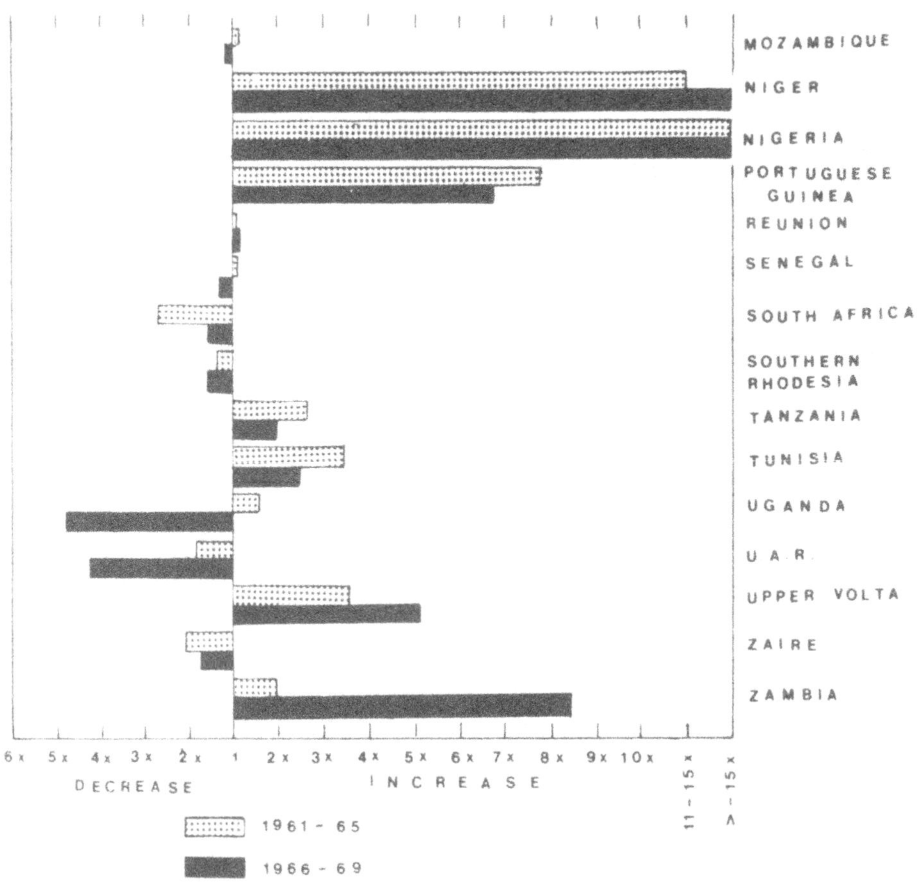

Fig. 1-b Changes in incidence of poliomyelitis in 31 African countries during the periods 1961-65 and 1966-69 as compared to 1951-55. (From Reference 4)

TABLE II

AVERAGE ANNUAL NUMBERS OF CASES - RELATION TO EFFECTIVE VACCINATION PROGRAMS

Area	Vaccination Programs	Cases of Poliomyelitis		
		1951-55	1961-65	1966-70
N. America, Europe, Australia and New Zealand	Effective and regular	72,737	7,517	789
4 Asian and 4 Central and South American Countries*	Effective and regular	3,623	893	78
Other Countries in Central and South America	Variable and irregular	4,023	3,759	3,038
35 African and Asian Countries	Mainly non-existent	2,393	6,779	7,777

*Cuba, Jamaica, Puerto Rico, Uruguay:
Hong Kong, Israel, Japan, Singapore

The fall in incidence in Europe, North America, etc. has already been discussed. The eight countries (four in Latin America and four in Asia) where a regular vaccination program has been carried out over a number of years also provide evidence of a considerable (and sustained) decrease. In contrast, the remaining countries listed in the table, and particularly those in Africa and Asia, show a very considerable increase in incidence.

I now wish to turn to an aspect of immunization with live polioviruses in countries with warm climates which has only relatively recently received detailed attention - the poor sero-conversion rates often found in children vaccinated in these areas. Let me first emphasize that live poliovirus vaccine, when properly used, gives good results in tropical areas.

In Table 3 is presented the sero-conversion rates after one dose of trivalent vaccine. In the warm climate countries, the percentage of "converters" varies greatly between countries and also between the virus types. Let us concentrate on type 1 which is epidemiologically the most important. The sero-conversion rates vary from 39 percent in Thailand (14) and Iran (13) to 87 percent in Costa Rica (10).

Apart from Tailand and Iran, however, the responses to type 1 are as good or better than those obtained in the Public Health Laboratory Service study in the United Kingdom in 1961 (19). In Iran the responses to all three types were poor and one may speculate whether the vaccine was still of good potency when it was administered.

In this same table are shown the concentrations of vaccine, whether only small numbers were vaccinated at a time or whether mass campaigns were made. The mass campaigns are divided into those carried out over a short period "S", or a long period "L". It is obvious that there were considerable variations in the dosage of vaccine but this is not correlated with the proportion of converters.

Dr. Sabin has frequently stressed the desirability of vaccination in tropical countries by mass campaigns completed in a matter of days. In this table the short-period campaigns gave better sero-conversion rates than the long-period campaigns.

In Table 4 is presented sero-conversion rates as a result of giving two or three doses of trivalent vaccine. With two doses, the rates for type 1 vary from 35 percent in a very carefully conducted study of small numbers of children in India (17) to 97 percent in the Costa Rica study (10) which also appears in the previous table.

Note that the best results with two doses were as good as the results with three doses in the United Kingdom. In South Africa (12) and Thailand (14) the results of three doses were also very good.

As in Table 3, the amounts of virus fed differed considerably in the different areas, but again there is no very clear correlation between virus concentration and serum conversion rates, and again there is an association between the type of mass campaign carried out - short or long period - and the percentage of converters. Thus, to stress the point once more, live poliovirus vaccines if properly administered in mass campaigns will give good epidemiological results. However, it is also apparent that in certain circumstances the serological results, and probably also the

TABLE III

SERO-CONVERSION RATES AFTER ONE DOSE OF TRIVALENT VACCINE

Country (and Reference)	Type of Campaign		Sero-conversion Rate (%)		
			Type 1	Type 2	Type 3
Costa Rica (10)	50% of children ≤ 13 years in one town	?S*	87[ns]	43[ns]	91[ns]
Mexico (11)	Mass	S	68[$10^{5.2-}_{5.6}$]ɵ	82[$10^{5.2-}_{5.6}$]	43[$10^{5.2-}_{5.6}$]
South Africa (12)	Mass	S	51[2-3x10^5]	87[2-3x10^5]	85[2-3x10^5]
Iran (13)	Mass	L+	39[3x10^5]	23[10^3]	36[10^5]
Thailand (14)	Small numbers in nurseries		39[10^6]	86[10^5]	65[3x10^5]
United Kingdom (19)	134 children living at home		54[10^6]	98[10^6]	48[10^6]

* Vaccination over a very short period

\+ Vaccination over a long period

ɵ Virus concentration

ns Not stated

TABLE IV

SERO-CONVERSION RATES AFTER MORE THAN ONE DOSE OF TRIVALENT VACCINE

Doses Given	Place (and Reference)	Type of Campaign		Sero-Conversion Rate (%)		
				Type 1	Type 2	Type 3
TWO	Costa Rica (10)	50% of children ≤ 13 years in one town	?S*	97[ns]$^{\theta}$	69[ns]	100[ns]
TWO	Mexico (11)	Mass	S	96[$10^{5.2-5.6}$]	96[$10^{5.2-5.6}$]	72[$10^{5.2-5.6}$]
TWO	South Africa (12)	Mass	S	93[2-3x10^5]	98[2-3x10^5]	99[2-3x10^5]
TWO	Bolivia (15)	Mass	L^+	87[$10^{5.3-5.7}$]	100[$10^{5.3-5.7}$]	96[$10^{5.3-5.7}$]
TWO	Iran (13) (Teheran)	Mass	L^+	79[3x10^5]	80[10^3]	75[10^5]
TWO	Thailand (14)	Small numbers in nurseries		77[10^6]	96[10^5]	97[3x10^5]
TWO	Hong Kong (16)	Mass	S	66[$10^{5.3}$]	99[$10^{5.3}$]	95[$10^{5.3}$]
TWO	Singapore (18)	Mass	L	50[$10^{5.3}$]	99[$10^{5.3}$]	59[$10^{5.3}$]
TWO	India (17)	200 children		35	77	47
THREE	South Africa (12)	Mass	S	100[2-3x10^5]	100[2-3x10^5]	100[2-3x10^5]
THREE	Thailand (14)	Small numbers		83[10^6]	100[10^5]	100[3x10^5]
THREE	United Kingdom(19)	Small numbers		97[10^6]	100[10^6]	99[10^6]

* Vaccination over a very short period; + Vaccination over a long period; θ Virus concentration
ns Not stated.

epidemiological results, will be considerably below expectation.

Various reasons for the phenomenon have been put forward:

1. Unsatisfactory storage and distribution of the vaccine;

2. Use of insensitive tests for measuring antibody;

3. Presence of local immunity due to previous contact with small doses of polioviruses or with other viruses;

4. Antibody in breast milk.

HANDLING AND STORAGE OF VACCINE

Examples of bad storage and handling of the vaccine are by no means unknown - even in Israel! - but Montefiore (9) has examined on several occasions batches of vaccine taken from the field during studies which have given poor ser-conversion rates and found them satisfactory. This is also true of the vaccines used in at least some of the studies above. Also, Montefiore (9) reports, "We have deliberately exposed samples of vaccine stabilized with magnesium chloride to more extreme conditions than could be expected to occur during actual use... and have found that the titer... remained satisfactory".

INSENSITIVE TESTS

This possibility has also been recently reviewed (9) and it is concluded that though there have been considerable variations in the methods of collecting blood samples, the starting dilutions of the sera, and in the types of test employed, however, the low sero-conversion rates cannot be accounted for on the basis of these differences.

INTERFERENCE

Interference from other enteroviruses was demonstrated early by a number of workers (18,21,22) and seemed a reasonable and satisfying explanation. However, other equally careful observers have failed to confirm these findings.

In the study by John and Jayabal (1,7) in Vellore, India, supported by WHO, about 200 children were fed vaccine (two doses at an eight-week interval) and samples of stool were collected at three weeks, two weeks and one week before vaccination, on the day each dose was given, and one week and two weeks after vaccination.

Samples from the specimens were inoculated into new-born mice, MK cells and Hep 2 cells. It was found that the sero-conversion rates for children excreting enteroviruses was 22 percent for type 1, 56 percent for type 2 and 30 percent for type 3. In children not excreting enteroviruses the corresponding rates were 14 percent for type 1, 54 percent for type 2 and 28 percent for type 3. Furthermore, no difference was observed between children excreting viruses in all the specimens obtained before vaccination and children with enteroviruses only in the specimen taken at the time the vaccine was given.

In this extremely careful study, therefore, the presence or absence of detectable enteroviruses did not influence the sero-conversion rates. However, Swartz and his colleagues in an equally careful study (also supported by WHO) have shown clear differences in sero-conversion rates and the geometric mean levels of antibody between excreters and non-excreters of enteroviruses - so obviously the matter is not yet settled.

LOCAL IMMUNITY

At an informal WHO meeting in Helsinki in 1968 (and indeed much earlier) Dr. Sabin put forward suggestions that local gut immunity due to repeated contact with small doses of polioviruses might explain some of the findings. Because of the obvious practical difficulties very little attempt has been made to examine this possibility. In any event, vaccine studies show that it is possible to obtain good serological responses by feeding vaccine repeatedly. It is also known that as a result of contact with natural poliovirus infections, the sero-conversion rates in tropical areas reach about 100 percent by the time children are three to five years old. The presence of local immunity does not therefore seem to be a probable explanation of the poor sero-conversion rates obtained in the vaccination program.

ANTIBODY IN BREAST MILK

It has been recognized that antibody can be present in breast milk since the studies by Sabin and his colleagues in the 1950's (23). These antibodies are capable of neutralizing live poliovirus for as long as 356 days after the birth of the child (24). A number of studies have shown that the antibody in milk (the level of which is roughly correlated with that of the serum) interferes with the take rates and sero-conversion rates, the degree of interference varying with the amount of antibody in the milk (25-27). However, the length of time over which this inhibitory effect persists has not been definitely determined. Warren and his colleagues (26) consider it safe to feed vaccine when the child is six weeks old in spite of the fact that antibody may still be present. Katz and Plotkin (27) and others have studied the effect of withholding breast feeding for varying periods before and after feeding the vaccine. With type 1, Katz and Plotkin (27) showed in children in Philadelphia that if there was no breast feeding for six hours before and six hours after vaccination, the take rates were very high. When the intervals were two hours before and two hours after, none of ten children were successfully vaccinated and when the intervals were two hours before and six hours after, or vice versa, the take rates were about 60 percent. Adcock and Green's (29) observations on children (also American) fed trivalent vaccine tend to confirm these findings.

Katz and Plotkin (27) suggest that boiled water should be given instead of the feed before and the feed after vaccination but Peradze *et al* (30) did not believe it was practicable in Nigeria to withhold breast feeding for more than half an hour or so.

There is obviously need for more observations in tropical areas before the exact importance of the inhibitory effect of antibody in breast milk can be assessed, and Dr. Dömök, Head of the WHO Virus Studies Team which is stationed at the East African Virus Research Institute, Entebbe, is currently investigating this question.

CONCLUSIONS

This review of the possible reasons for less than optimal sero-conversion rates which are sometimes (but not always) obtained after the use of live vaccine in the tropics leaves us, unfortunately, unable to say which of the four factors mentioned may be the most important. Perhaps there are also other factors, for example malnutrition or genetic differences.

However, as mass vaccination with two or three doses of trivalent vaccine gives a satisfactory epidemiological result in most instances you may ask why so much stress should be laid on the question. One reason is that an understanding of the different responses in tropical and temperate-climate children may well improve our knowledge of the non-humoral mechanisms of immunity. But of more immediate practical importance is the fact that as time goes on mass immunization campaigns will gradually cease to be acceptable to health authorities and immunization will become merged into the general public health services as these develop and improve.

It is thus essential to ensure that the best possible vaccine will be available when the time comes for vaccination programs in developing countries to be organized on the same lines as those in developed countries - when only relatively small numbers of children will be presented for vaccination at any one time, and when according to present evidence the vaccine is likely to be put to the most stringent tests of its immunizing potency.

REFERENCES

1. DROZDOV, S.G. & COCKBURN, W.C. Pan American Health Organization *Scientific Publication No. 147:*198, 1967.
2. COCKBURN, W.C. & DROZDOV, S.G. *Bull. World Health Org. 42:* 405, 1970.
3. DROZDOV, S.G. & COCKBURN, W.C. Pan American Health Organization *Scientific Publication No. 226:*163, 1971.
4. DÖMÖK, I. Recent Progress in Immunization: Poliomyelitis, Given at the Seminar on Immunization in Africa, organized by the International Children's Centre, Paris, in Kampala, 1971 (unpublished data)
5. CHASTEL, C. *Rev. Hyg. Med. Soc. 17:*367, 1969.
6. PERABO, F.E. *Lancet II:*926, 1970.
7. SABIN, A.B. *Trop. Geogr. Med. 15:*38, 1963.
8. The Second Ten Years of the World Health Organization, WHO, Geneva, p. 18, 1968.
9. MONTEFIORE, D. Pan American Health Organization *Scientific Publication No. 226:*182, 1971.
10. ROCA-GARCIA, M. ET AL. *J. Am. Med. Ass. 188:*639, 1964.
11. SABIN, A.B. ET AL. *J. Am. Med. Ass. 173:*1521, 1960.
12. WINTER, P.A.D. ET AL. *S. Afr. Med. J. 37:*510, 1963.
13. NATEGH, R. ET AL. *Trop. Geogr. Med. 22:*303, 1970.
14. SANGKAWIBHA, N. ET AL. *J. Med. Ass. Thailand 52:*701, 1969.
15. GUACHALLA, G.J. ET AL. *Rev. Salud Publ. Boliviana IV 19:*25, 1963.
16. FRANKLIN, G.C. & ROBERTSON, M.J. *Pub. Health (Lond.) 79:*81, 1965.
17. JOHN, T.J. & JAYABAL, P. (To be published.)
18. LEE, L.H. ET AL. *Brit. Med. J. i:*1077, 1964.
19. Report of the Public Health Laboratory Service, *Brit. Med. J. ii:*1037, 1961.
20. SWARTZ, T.A., SKALSKA, P., GERICHTER, C.A. & COCKBURN, W.C. (To be published.)
21. RAMOS ALVAREZ, M. Pan American Health Organization *(Scientific Publication No. 147:*213, 1967.
22. MONTEFIORE, D.G., JAMIESON, M.J., COLLARD, P. & JOLLY, H. *Brit. Med. J. i:*1569, 1963.
23. SABIN, A.B. *WHO Monograph No. 26:*297, 1955.
24. SABIN, A.B. & FIELDSTEEL, A.H. *Pediatrics 29:*105, 1962.
25. SABIN, A.B., MICHAELS, R.H. KRUGMAN, S., EIGER, M.E., BERMAN, P.H. & WARREN, J. *Pediatrics 31:*623, 1963.

26. WARREN, R.J., LEPOW, M.L., BARTSCH, G.E. & ROBBINS, F.C. *Pediatrics 34*:4, 1964.
27. KATZ, M. & PLOTKIN, S.A. *J. Pediat. 73*:267, 1968.
28. PLOTKIN, S.A., KATZ, M., BROWN, R.E. & REGANO, J.S. *Am. J. Dis. Child. 111*:27, 1966.
29. ADCOCK, E. & GREENE, H. *Lancet II*:662, 1971.
30. PERADZE, T., MONTEFIORE, D. & COKER, G. *W. Afr. Med. J. 17*:122, 1968.

NON-POLIO VIRUS INTERFERENCE WITH ORAL POLIO VACCINE IMMUNIZATION: POSSIBLE INFLUENCE OF PHYSICAL CLIMATE AND SOCIO-ECONOMIC STATUS

T. A. Swartz[1], Paulina Skalska[2], C. B. Gerichter[2], and W. C. Cockburn[3]

Department of Clinical Epidemiology, Asaf Harofe Hospital, Tel Aviv University Medical School, Zerifin, Beer Yaakov, Israel[1]

In spite of the widespread use of oral polio vaccine (O.P.V.), vaccination programs in many tropical and subtropical countries have apparently failed to provide the expected results in the control of paralytic poliomyelitis (1). Among several factors considered responsible for these unsatisfactory results, an important role has been attributed to the interferences of naturally occurring enteroviral infections on the "take rate" in the intestine, following O.P.V. administration (2,3).

Since the risk of exposure to agents of acute gastrointestinal infections, including enteroviruses, is associated with, among other factors, the season, particularly the hot season, and the socio-economic status (4), it was of interest to investigate the effect of O.P.V. administered at different times of the year to different socio-economic groups living in a warm climate, such as pertains in Israel.

MATERIAL AND METHODS

Infants from the Tel-Aviv and Ashdod areas, two months old at the start of the study, were routinely administered O.P.V. at the age of two, four and six months, in two trials, performed in winter and summer. The infants were categorized into two socio-economic groups (high and low).

[2]Central Virologic Laboratory, Ministry of Health, Jaffa, Israel

[3]Virus Diseases, WHO, Geneva,Switzerland

Virologic and serologic tests were carried out on fecal and serum samples collected before and after each of the O.P.V. administrations. Fecal excretion of non-polio virus (N.P.V.), indicative of potential interference, was studied in the week following O.P.V. administration.

RESULTS

Table 1 indicates the relationship between polio immunization, expressed as percent of seroconversion and geometric mean (G.M.) level of neutralizing antibody, and the presence of N.P.V. in fecal excretion.

In infants who did not excrete N.P.V., only slight differences in the percent of seroconversion and G.M. level of polio antibody are observed between the two social groups in both seasons; in the case where N.P.V. is excreted, seroconversion rates and G.M. levels in both social groups are distinctly lower in summer than in winter, with the lowest values occurring in the summer-fed low social groups.

COMMENTS

Many previous studies in warm climates indicate a poor polio seroconversion in the presence of high rates of N.P.V. excretion (3-6). The same trend was recently observed in a study carried out in a rather cold climate (7).

The significant differences in the seroconversion rates and G.M. antibody level between N.P.V. excretors and non-excretors in the summer trial indicate an association between the presence of N.P.V. excretion, the tendency to lower polio immunity and the higher summer temperature. The quite striking difference between the two social groups attests to a contributory role of the lower socio-economic status in hindering the immunity process (8,9).

High rates of excretion of N.P.V. occurring together with unsatisfactory rates of polio seroconversion and low G.M. levels suggest interference of non-polio enteroviruses with replication of O.P.V. viruses in the gut of the vaccinees. The summer preeminence of this phenomenon in both socio-economic groups, but particularly in the lower one, emphasizes the roles of both the climatic factor and the social environment in altering the polio immunity of segments of the population with low standards of personal hygiene, by increasing their exposure to intestinal virus infections.

TABLE I

RELATIONSHIP BETWEEN POLIO NEUTRALIZING ANTIBODY AND NON-POLIO VIRUS EXCRETION

Study Group	Distribution of Polio Neutralizing Antibody											
	Without Non-Polio Virus Excretion						With Non-Polio Virus Excretion					
	Type 1		Type 2		Type 3		Type 1		Type 2		Type 3	
	%	G.M.*	%	G.M.	%	G.M.	%	G.M.	%	G.M.	%	G.M.
Winter												
High Social Group	100.0	127	100.0	151	100.0	151	100.0	108	100.0	160	100.0	108
Low Social Group	100.0	116	100.0	147	97.0	118	100.0	108	100.0	108	100.0	108
Summer												
High Social Group	95.0	109	100.0	149	100.0	149	83.3	45	100.0	127	83.3	45
Low Social Group	94.1	102	100.0	160	94.1	129	50.0	20	83.3	61	65.0	30

*Geometric mean antibody level.

CONCLUSIONS

Unsatisfactory immunization of the low socio-economic group given O.P.V. appeared to be associated, in our summer trial, with non-polio enterovirus interference.

REFERENCES

1. COCKBURN, W.C. & DROZDOV, S.G. *Bull. World Health Org.* *42:* 405, 1970.
2. HORSTMAN, D. *The Med. Clinics of N. Am.* *61:*681, 1967.
3. SABIN, A.B. Poliomyelitis. Accomplishments of Live Virus Vaccine. In: Proceedings of First International Conf. on Vaccines Against Viral and Rickettsial Diseases of Man, p. 17, Washington, D.C., Pan American Health Org. 1967.
4. RAMOS-ALVAREZ, M. Section A in: *Ibid.,* p. 213.
5. DROZDOV, S. & COCKBURN, W.C. Poliomyelitis in the Developed and Developing Countries, In: Conference on the Application of Vaccines Against Viral, Rickettsial and Bacterial Diseases of Man, p. 163, Washington, D.C., Pan American Health Org., 1971.
6. MONTEFIORE, D.G. Problems of Poliomyelitis Immunization in Countries with Warm Climate. In: *Ibid.,* p. 182.
7. Scottish Home and Health Department. Communicable Diseases, Scotland, Weekly Report 71/39, 11, 1971.
8. PORTLAND, D.J., PLEXICO, K., FLYNT, W. & CHIN, T.D.Y. *Pub. Health Rep.* *83:*507, 1968.
9. MILLAR, E.C.M. *Pub. Health Rep.* *85:*1036, 1971.

ROUND TABLE CONFERENCE

Members of the Panel:

H.G. Pereira, Chairman

P. Biggs, P. Brunell , C. Cockburn, V. Cabasso,
I. Gresser, M. Sela

Pereira: Four questions will be debated at this Round Table Discussion: The current need for vaccines; vaccines against cancer; the advantages and disadvantages of the use of subunit vaccines; and how can one improve the immunogenicity of vaccines.

As regards the first topic, it has been mentioned that some vaccines are more needed than others. Some that proved useful in the past are now in less demand as the respective diseases come under control. There are cases where it is difficult to decide whether a particular vaccine is worthwhile developing or not. While pondering these questions, we shall also consider vaccines against cancer. A broader view of the subject will bring into consideration also treatments other than vaccination in the prevention and control of viral diseases and cancer, such as passive immunity by administration of antibodies, the use of non-specific measures such as interferon, etc.

Let us ask, what vaccines are needed? In our work, we have been concerned with adenovirus. The need for adenovirus vaccine is a debatable point. Not everyone agrees that such a vaccine is necessary. The epidemiologists and pediatricians may have something to say about this.

Cabasso: No doubt, great improvements will be made in the viral vaccines of the future. Subunit vaccines, or vaccines containing only the relevant antigen, highly purified or even in crystalline form, will become available for routine use. One can even hope that the images so tantilizingly evoked by Dr. Arnon when she discussed synthetic vaccines will become reality some day.

Realistically, though, need for a vaccine is not established mainly on the basis that the vaccine is already developed. For example, the availability of a purified, crystalline hexon antigen for adenovirus type 5 is not reason enough to decide that it is needed for mass immunization.

Those of us charged with the development of vaccines needed for protection against present threats often must meet the need for given vaccines with less than ideal immunogens. Serious consideration must also be given to three broad areas, or groups of factors, before a decision can be made to undertake the development of a vaccine. These groups or factors are:

1. epidemiological factors;
2. factors concerned with pathogenesis;
3. factors involved with feasibility.

1. Epidemiologic factors:

Among the factors related to epidemiology are the incidence and severity of the disease, and the climatic, environmental and socio-economic conditions under which it occurs. A clear illustration is found in the application of oral poliomyelitis vaccine: whereas colonization of the gut is readily achieved with this vaccine in cold and temperate zones, it is less easily obtained in warm climates where infection of the intestine with other enteroviruses is prevalent. But incidence and severity are of even more fundamental importance.

a. Incidence: The need for mass vaccination varies greatly even among widespread infections. Mass vaccination is certainly greatly needed against poliomyelitis, yellow fever, the common cold and viral hepatitis, for example. Vaccines against poliomyelitis and yellow fever have become available, but none is yet available against the common cold or viral hepatitis.

   In other widespread infections, the need for vaccination may not be as apparent. An example of this would be adenovirus infection of humans: whereas vaccination of military recruits against certain adenovirus serotypes was found necessary, that of civilian populations is not being recommended despite the wide circulation of this class of viruses.

   The problem takes on a differen aspect when sporadic infections are considered. A case in point is that of viral encephalitis in the U.S.A. Acute outbreaks have occurred from time to time, with loss of twenty or more lives in some. Yet vaccination of the entire population is considered unrealistic and, even though feasible, no vaccine specifically intended for humans has been developed. It is fortunate that the spread of these infections can effectively be interrupted by the use of insecticides.

Finally, some infections, although endangering only few individuals, were rated as deserving of attention and of the efforts to develop vaccines for their control. They concern most laboratory workers, and Venezuelan equine encephalitis and herpes B virus infections belong in this category.

b. Severity: Even though its incidence in humans may be limited, the extent to which a disease is disabling greatly influences the level of efforts made to control it. Herpes B virus infection is one against which a great deal of energy was invested in the development of a vaccine. Rabies is another low incidence disease which, because of its fatality, brought about the first vaccine ever developed by man for deliberate protection against an inevitable death.

When disabling effect is combined with high incidence, the problem becomes more acute. Adenovirus infection in the military illustrates well this point: because of the severe lower respiratory involvement and the resulting loss of manpower due to this disease, adenovirus vaccines are of high priority among military authorities.

At times, attitudes toward the necessity of controlling a viral infection change as knowledge about it increases. Rubella was considered as a widespread but inconsequential indisposition of childhood, not requiring prevention. But when the potential damaging effect of the virus on the gestating fetus was discovered, concerted and intense efforts to develop a vaccine were undertaken.

But alas, there are still a number of widespread and severe, or highly incommodating diseases against which there is as yet no vaccine development, despite the great need and the considerable effort invested. Such is the case with viral hepatitis and the common cold.

2. Factors Concerned with Pathogenesis:

Elements such as portal of entry, CNS involvement, teratogenesis and other factors influence the choice of approach in vaccine development, and the very chances of success.

a. Portal of entry: Only because poliovirus invades the susceptible subject via the oral cavity, is acid-resistant, and multiplies in the intestine, is oral poliomyelitis vaccine the success it turned out to be. When the same vaccine was deliberately or inadvertently injected subcutaneously or intramuscularly, it induced no detectable sero-immunity, unless the vaccine virus found its way to the intestinal mucosa.

   So far, experience with oral immunization against some myxo-like viruses, whose portal of entry is the respiratory mucosa, has not been very encouraging. This is not too surprising, as these viruses would be inactivated by the gastric acid. Furthermore, it is doubtful that they would multiply to the required extent in the intestine, as suggested by the poor results obtained with enteric-coated preparations.

   Another very successful vaccine, that against yellow fever, is administered parenterally, the route by which the infection is transmitted in nature by the mosquito. It is not always possible, however, to use the natural pathway of a viral infection for vaccination purposes. In some cases, the attenuated virus may not have retained the invasiveness of its natural counterpart, as was experienced with the Edmonston strain of measles virus and the HPV77 rubella virus when administered by the respiratory route. In others, the practice may not be without risk, as would be the inhalation of vaccinating virus, for example. In these circumstances, and particularly with inactivated viral vaccines, the parenteral route is ordinarily resorted to, regardless of the portal of entry.

b. CNS involvement: When a virus disease syndrome includes significant involvement of the CNS, it is particularly essential that a potential vaccine against it be scrutinized for any residual affinity for nervous tissue. This was a most critical step in the development of poliomyelitis, measles and mumps vaccines, and in that of live, attenuated rabies vaccines for dogs, cats and cattle.

c. Teratogenicity: In domestic animals in nature, a number of viruses can invade the fetus, and cause abortion and/or malformation. Among those are infectious bovine rhinotracheitis virus, bluetongue virus of sheep and hog cholera virus. Although effective, live, attenuated vaccines were developed against these viruses, their teratogenic effect was not abolished and in practice they are not recommended for the vaccination of dams at certain stages of gestation.

A very similar experience was observed with rubella virus, the most notorious teratogenic virus in man: although rubella vaccine was demonstrated safe and effective in children and non-pregnant adults, the vaccine virus was found capable of invading the fetus in early pregnancy.

d. Other involvements: One of the clearest examples of the importance to know as much as possible about the pathogenesis of a disease in vaccine development is the varicella-Herpes Zoster complex. Like rubella, varicella is ordinarily a mild disease of childhood, but while CNS involvement is practically absent in rubella, it may occur in varicella. But more seriously, unlike rubella, the varicella virus continues to reside in latent form in the host after recovery, and may reappear later as Herpes Zoster. The dilemma which is faced when considering a vaccine against varicella can be summed up as follows: a killed vaccine would in all probability be inadequate, as it may require multiple and periodic administration; on the other hand, a live, attenuated virus may also reside in the recipient in latent form, and later in life perhaps be triggered to cause Zoster. A lifetime may be needed to establish the safety of a live varicella vaccine.

At times, incomplete knowledge of the immunopathology of a disease may lead to vaccines more damaging than the diseases proper. For example, use of an inactivated respiratory syncytial (RS) vaccine in infants did elicit formation of circulating antibody, but when exposure to the natural virus occurred, the disease induced in the vaccinated children was more severe than in those unvaccinated. Retrospectively, this exacerbation was not deemed unexpected, as severe forms of the disease were observed most frequently in infants with maternal antibody. This led to the hypothesis that the disease caused by RS virus is due to a reaction of virus-antibody complex at the level of the alveoli - an Arthus-type reaction.

Further, it was found that IgG is not protective in RSV, and that only IgA in the nasal mucosa could prevent invasion by RSV via the nasal route. The prospects for a successful vaccination against RSV now reside in the development of a live, attenuated virus which would be administered intranasally.

3. Factors Involved with Feasibility:

Last but not least are the factors related to feasibility of vaccine development. These include the avenues available for deliberate prophylaxis, the etiology of the disease, methods of propagation of the virus and substrates to be used, demonstration of safety and efficacy, and purely economic factors.

It is essential at first to explore the type of prophylactic approach to be taken. In arbovirus infections, for example, destruction of the insect-vector may be the method of control of choice.

If immunization is the more logical avenue to consider, should it be of the passive or active type? If a vaccine is to be employed, must it be live, attenuated, or could a potent, inactivated vaccine accomplish the desired result?

Whatever the type of vaccine wanted, it is necessary that the etiological agent of the disease be isolated and clearly identified, and that the number of sero-types of the virus be determined. Furthermore, rich cultures of the virus or viruses must be made readily available. In recent years, the advent of tissue culture has greatly increased feasibility in this regard, but a series of practical problems relating to virus yield, stability, purification, concentration, inactivation if necessary, and tests for safety and potency must first be solved. There are, in addition, problems of a more theoretical nature that are less easily solved, and for some of these there is no precedent to provide guidance. These problems are concerned primarily with safety and include: the kind of cell cultures acceptable for vaccine preparation, freedom from extraneous viruses, possible adverse effects from the administration of the vaccine virus itself, and the safety of "immunoadjuvants" that may have to be used.

Proof of the protective efficacy of a vaccine is relatively simple to obtain in diseases that occur in epidemics or have generally high attack rates, such as influenza or adenovirus infection. This is also the case in illnesses that are readily diagnosed clinically, such as measles. But in diseases such as those due to parainfluenza or respiratory syncytial viruses, the clinical features of which are not pathognomonic, vaccines against individual viruses may appear to have little effect on the total incidence of respiratory disease. Evaluation of these vaccines, therefore, requires new approaches. The correlation of the presence of antibody and protection can at times be established in experimental animals, and sero-conversion can serve later as an index of efficacy in man. Controlled, deliberate challenge of human volunteers may have to be resorted to, in certain cases, providing the risks involved are low.

Finally, economic factors also play an important role in the development of viral vaccines. Incidence of the disease, the potential demand for and the extent of application of a vaccine against it, the estimated cost of research and development, all are questions that are looked into carefully before launching on a program of vaccine development.

It goes without saying that the importance of these factors varies according to the disease under consideration. It is high in the case of diseases of domestic animals which constitute a threat to human welfare or life, but diminishes in that of other zoonoses or human diseases according to the risk involved. For example, great efforts have been put into the protection of laboratory workers against some of the exotic diseases they may be investigating, even though the demand for a vaccine may in such instances be low. On the other hand, economics are in great measure responsible for the relatively few improvements introduced into human rabies vaccine since the days of Pasteur.

Recently uncovered virus diseases present greater complexities than older ones, and chances of developing effective vaccines against some are more remote. These problems require the attention not only of expert virologists and immunologists, but also of experimental clinicians and specialists in epidemiology. The facilities required for undertaking the study of these diseases are also quite elaborate, and all those requirements constitute a heavy financial burden. Many such projects are no longer within the reach of the private sector of our economy, and governments have to step in to fill the needs and expend necessarily large sums of money. The U.S. Government, for example, has had to finance the development of a number of human and animal virus vaccines.

In conclusion, then, it is not always sufficient to have available purified antigens to justify embarking on mass prophylaxis programs; the many factors detailed above have also to be reckoned with. No wonder that the list of available vaccines shown yesterday by Dr. Beale is relatively modest, in the face of the large number of viral infections which remain to be conquered.

Brunell: I should like to focus your attention on the herpes group of viruses. We now recognize a number of herpes viruses that produce disease in the human species.

1. Herpes type 1 is associated with a syndrome of ulcerative lesions of the oral mucosa, and high fever in infancy and childhood; recrudescences later result in "cold sores" which may be incapacitating in some individuals.

2. Herpes type 2 has been associated but not etiologically linked to cervical cancer. This virus also produces severe morbidity in infants born through an infected birth canal. These babies develop disseminated disease.

3. Cytomegalovirus (CMV) may cause mental retardation. It has been estimated that about 1 percent of children (30,000/year) born in the U.S.A. are infected with CMV at birth and about 10 percent of them develop some mental deficiency (3,000).

4. Infectious mononucleosis virus was first identified in Burkitt's lymphoma cell cultures (EB virus). Whether this virus is etiologically related to Burkitt's lymphoma is unsettled as yet.

5. The last group which has been recognized thus far is varicella-zoster (V-Z) virus.

Let us consider varicella-zoster virus as a prototype for a herpes virus vaccine. If one considers the natural history of v.z.v. infection, we recognize that it occurs in children and produces very little morbidity; most individuals are infected during childhood. After clinical recovery from this infection, the virus persists in the human host in a latent form, i.e., in the absence of clinical disease. At some time, perhaps decades later, this latent virus may become activated and produce zoster or "shingles". This condition produces a considerable amount of morbidity in aged persons. In some individuals, particularly in immunosuppressed patients, zoster may become generalized and produce a life-threatening illness.

If a live virus vaccine is produced against v.z.v., its efficacy (as with any other live attenuated vaccine), must be assessed by considering the morbidity produced by the vaccine, as compared to that produced by the natural infection.

In the case of v.z.v. or any other attenuated latent viruses, the problem of activation of latent virus (zoster) must be considered. It would be necessary, therefore, to be able to observe our vaccinees for a period of decades in order to be sure that we have not selected a strain of virus for the vaccine that would produce more frequent or more severe zoster than what would be expected following natural infection.

Since patients with zoster provide a natural reservoir of virus which can then infect the rest of the population it would be difficult to eradicate this virus from the population. Those individuals who did not obtain this vaccine early in life would grow to adulthood susceptible to v-z infection. They then might be exposed to this reservoir of infection and get varicella at a time of life when the disease would be much more severe than if they had contracted it in childhood when it is a relatively mild disease.

Cockburn: The questions which should be answered when one discusses the necessity of vaccines are:

1. How to influence the disease in a population and bring it down to a manageable size;

2. How long can one leave between vaccinations?

3. What can be done about combination and simultaneous administrations of virus vaccines?

With the number of vaccines we have available at the moment, proper use within the next ten years would enormously change the whole morbidity situation and free the population of the world from a number of communicable diseases.

In this connection I should like to mention the pertussis vaccine. Effective pertussis vaccines can and are being prepared, but it is easy for their potency to decline. In addition, reactions to the vaccine often cause concern. Nevertheless, in recent years, no one has made serious attempts to look at the structure of the pertussis bacillus and to isolate non-reactive effective subunit vaccines.

When one thinks of new vaccines that might be required, one immediately thinks of herpes vaccines. Another really serious, world-wide problem, is infectious hepatitis and if a vaccine against it were available, it would be of enormous importance.

Brunell: I should like to add to the list of needed vaccines also that against viral diarrhoea; this problem has not received yet sufficient attention from virologists.

Viral gastroenteritis accounts for considerable morbidity in underdeveloped nations; it is also one of the leading causes of death in childhood in more advanced countries.

Cabasso: Although means to develop ideal immunogens are not at hand in most instances, the pursuit of purified subunit virus vaccines must be continued without abatement wherever possible. Some problems, however, demand more immediate attention; and passive immunization may provide some solutions.

For instance, we do not have very satisfactory rabies vaccines for the protection of man. Present vaccines are crude preparations of variable antigenicity, and effort is still being invested to improve them. It is readily admitted that today's vaccines are not totally effective in post-exposure immunization, particularly in cases of severe exposure: the time between exposure and irreversible engagement of the rabies virus in body tissues may be as short as a few hours or a few days. With present vaccines (14 or 21 daily injections) it may take as long as 9 - 11 days after the first injection before neutralizing antibody is detected, perhaps too late to effectively block progress of the virus. In such cases, passive immunization has provided an effective answer. Originally, the preformed antibody was of equine origin and not without undesirable side effects: as many as 30 percent of persons who received it developed serum sickness. Recently, therefore, efforts were made to substitute horse serum by rabies hyperimmune human gamma globulin, and success has been achieved. This, then, is an example of a situation where passive immunization is effective.

Another infection where passive immunization may prove of value, in the absence of other means of prophylaxis, is viral hepatitis B. Human gamma globulin having a high titer against Australia (hepatitis B) antigen has been prepared, and is at present being tested in cases of recent exposure - either by "needle stick" or through transfusion.

Other hyperimmune human gamma globulins which may prove beneficial under specified circumstances are under development against rubella and varicella-zoster. Dr. Brunnell will comment on the latter in greater detail.

Sela: With reference to Cabasso's remark about replacing animal antibodies by human antibodies, I would like to remind you that in the intact gamma globulin the most immuno-competent areas are situated in the Fc portion of the molecule. Even in the human gamma globulin, the potentionally most dangerous area is Fc. The Fc portion of the IgG molecule may be removed by enzymatic (e.g., pepsin, papain) or chemical (mild treatment with cyanogen bromides) means*.

---

* Cahnemann *et al*, J. Biol. Chem. 241:3247, 1966; Lahav *et al*, J. Exp. Med. 125:787, 1967.

When we remove this fragment, then regions of Fab which were before immunosilent, become immunopotent, but still Fab is definitely less immunogenic than the complete IgG molecule. It thus seems that it will be safer to use an animal or human globulin when one removes this one third which is useless immunologically as a vaccine since it does not contain combining sites, but is dangerous because it may create additional immunological problems.

Brunell: I should like to raise the problem of passive immunization in the immuno-suppressed patient. There are patients who are congenitally immunodeficient, and a growing number of individuals who are receiving immunosuppressive drugs for transplantation and treatment of various disorders. In both instances, these patients may not respond to standard vaccines.

We have been particularly concerned with varicella since patients who are immuno-suppressed suffer greater morbidity than do normal patients. In such cases passive immunization is advisable. Plasma from patients with zoster is fractionated and gamma globulin prepared from this material is given to high risk and immuno-suppressed patients, to protect them against infection at the time they are exposed.

Gresser: I am a believer in interferon for the following reasons: There are two theoretical objections that have been raised against the use of interferon:

1. It is prophylactic only;
2. The amounts required preclude its use as an active therapeutic substance.

In animal studies (using mice) neither statement is valid.

Let us consider the effect of interferon on a disease initiated by an infectious, virulent virus such as encephalomyocarditis (EMC) in mice. This virus kills all the mice within four to five days after infection. However, if one inoculates viral infected mice at daily intervals with interferon beginning 12 - 24 hours after injection of the virus, 75 percent of mice survive even when the infectious dose is of the order of 100 LD_{50}.

This is an example of what can be obtained in an acute viral infection. Similar results are obtained in a subacute viral disease, such as observed in mice inoculated with Rauscher leukemia virus. One can infect mice with this virus and then wait till symptoms of disease appear, for example a palpable spleen. If at this stage one administers exogenous interferon repeatedly, further manifestations of the disease are delayed and survival of animals is markedly increased. Also, in the spontaneous leukemia of AKR mice, repeated injections of interferon markedly increase the survival of mice.

In terms of cancer: One can inoculate mice with transplantable tumors of viral or non-viral origin - either in an ascitic form or as a subcutaneous solid tumor. For example, after inoculation of 10^4 Ehrlich ascites cells into a mouse - (one cell can kill a mouse) - one can wait for several days postinoculation and only then begin to treat these mice with interferon. Ninety percent of the mice are cured.

In fact, we have found in our laboratory that interferon is as potent, if not more potent, than the standard antitumor chemotherapeutic substances used. We use a 3 L L tumor which after subcutaneous inoculation gives rise with three weeks to metastatic foci in the lungs. Six days after the inoculation of tumor cells into mice, at a time when palpable subcutaneous nodules have appeared, daily inoculation of interferon will inhibit further development of the subcutaneous tumors and inhibit the appearance of metastatic foci.

I should stress that we have never observed any toxicity in mice treated with interferon.

The results of experimentation in animals with exogenous interferon are sufficiently promising to hope for its successful use in man. Even small amounts of exogenous interferon have therapeutic effects in mice infected with oncogenic or non-oncogenic viruses or inoculated with transplantable tumor cells.

As to the amounts of interferon needed: when one extrapolates from data obtained from tissue cultures, the amounts of interferon which should be effective in animals are much higher than those experimentally observed. Surprisingly small amounts of interferon were found to be effective *in vivo*. The exogenous interferon is also superior to the inducers of endogenous interferon, although inducers cause the production of greater amounts of endogenous interferon than the amounts achieved by injection of exogenous interferon.

Biggs: We heard from Hilleman that animal models exist in which vaccines have been used against both DNA and RNA tumor viruses. One has to bear in mind, however, that cancer is not a single disease. Therefore, when speaking of vaccines for human cancer, one needs to think in terms of multiple, or at best, polyvalent vaccines.

Then we encounter the real difficulty in choosing between live and killed vaccines. Can one ever envisage a live vaccine against cancer in man that could be acceptable? There are great difficulties in safety testing of such a vaccine. If we consider herpes viruses which at present are the most likely candidates for a vaccine, there is the example of herpes viruses which are innocuous in some species of monkey but oncogenic in others. It would be difficult to be sure that an experimental animal will show up the oncogenic potential for man of a human herpes virus such as E.B. virus.

A more acceptable idea, therefore, is the possibility of using killed vaccines. Turning to the other likely candidates for a human tumor virus, the C-type RNA viruses, we again need to learn from animal models. We need to assess the relative significance of vertical transmission and tolerance, and horizontal transmission, before consideration is given to the possibility of vaccines against these viruses.

There are many other problems which there is not time to discuss; however, if vaccines against cancer in man are to be considered, the first requirement, after the identification of a putative human tumor virus, is the finding of a suitable experimental host, or hosts, for safety and efficacy testing.

If killed vaccines are suggested, perhaps we should think of vaccines against antigen in tumor cell membranes rather than against structural viral proteins.

Pereira: Considering the parallel between Marek's disease (as a virus that has been controlled by a vaccine) and Burkitt's lymphoma in man, and that there is a virus that is associated with Burkitt's lymphoma, if it were possible to produce enough EB virus so as to make purified protein from it and use this for vaccination of a susceptible population, if such vaccination were safe then the results would indicate whether there is an etiological relationship between EBV and Burkitt's lymphoma.

Hilleman: Considering the incidence of Burkitt's lymphoma - in order to be able to assess the efficacy of such a vaccine one would have to vaccinate about 50,000 people in such a trial.

Biggs: The question would still remain what subunit of EB virus to use, and to know what are the virus-associated antigens which might be of importance. Secondly, there are no good techniques yet to grow these viruses in adequate quantities for this approach.

Cockburn: The time has come when large scale vaccination trials are not always feasible for the following reasons:

1. because the incidence of the disease may be too small to justify large scale trials;

2. because of uncertainty about the effects of vaccination;

3. because of problems of national policies.

It seems to me therefore, that analysis should be done by immunologists, who should first study the antibody response so as to indicate whether the vaccine is likely to be effective. To give an example: In Korea in two years we vaccinated 80,000 children (with another 80,000 participating as controls) in a study of killed vaccine of Japanese encephalitis - but there were no cases of this disease at all.

Hilleman: There are two approaches to be considered in the area of prophylaxis and treatment of cancer by immunologic procedures. The first of these is by immunization against infection with oncogenic viruses or by immunization against viruses which function as co-factors or inducers of oncogenesis by unrelated oncogenic viruses. The second of these is by immunizing against the unique antigens which are part of tumor cells.

Preparation of vaccines against cancer is a tough problem. It is not feasible today to prepare cancer virus vaccines for man because we do not have proved viruses which cause cancer in man. Until we get them, we shall have to content ourselves with work on animal cancer models. There are presently eight RNA and DNA viruses which are candidates as causative agents in human cancer. None is proved but foremost among them is the herpes simplex 2 virus which might be implicated in human cervical carcinoma.

Once the candidate viruses are proved, one might employ live or killed virus vaccine approaches. There are two points I think we should keep in mind. One of these is that our target should be to prevent the clinical expression of cancer. I don't think we can expect to prevent, totally, infection with oncogenic agents. If, however, we can limit infection or otherwise prevent the expression of infection as cancer, then the target objective is attained. The other matter is that naturally attenuated avirulent non-oncogenic counterparts of human oncogenic viruses should present the best approach to effective prophylaxis from the standpoint of efficacy and from the standpoint of license for use granted by the regulatory agencies. Turkey herpesvirus vaccine for prevention of Marek's disease of chickens is a prime example.

Tumor cell antigen vaccines have their greatest hope for use in treating cancer, once established, by enhancing immunologic resistance. This is an approach on which we have been working for more than a decade with the hope of isolating tumor specific antigens free of normal cell antigens. We feel it essential to remove, as much as possible, normal cell components so as to limit the risk of inducing auto-immune disease.

Goldblum: It seems to me that the concept of vaccination against cancer is still immature. Unless we know exactly the mechanism of cell transformation and tumor formation, we are still far from making good educated guesses about vaccines. Marek's disease is probably an exception. The use of virus vaccines made of oncogenic viruses should not theoretically do any good because of what is happening in the body. During viral infection, viral coat proteins are formed. If we want to prevent the formation of tumors there is no use in making antibodies against virus coat proteins. The use of purified antigens derived from cells, or cell walls - as previously indicated by Hilleman - may be at the moment the best answer to prevention of cancer.

Questions:

1. What is the interpretation of the role of interferon in the prevention of expression of cancer?

2. What is the state of the art in large-scale production of human interferon? Are monkeys still the source?

Gresser: Interferon is not exclusively an antiviral substance although it was discovered by virologists. It has a number of other biological effects, due to the molecule of interferon itself.

There are several interpretations of the mode of action of interferon in tumor prevention or therapy:

1. Inhibition of virus replication in spontaneous leukemia, e.g., vertically transmitted natural leukemias, thus reducing the chances of expression of cancer;

2. Interferon has a direct effect on the multiplication of the tumor cells once they develop;

3. Interferon may have an effect on host mechanisms of defence and may aid in the rejection of the tumor itself or in its inhibition.

Hilleman: Based on our own work, the estimated cost of making a single dose of safe and effective interferon would appear prohibitive in the practical sense. Not all would agree with this assessment and there are those who are pursuing the matter of exogenous interferon with practical hopes in mind.

As to the problem of prevention of cancer by vaccination, viral vaccines have been proved effective against RNA and DNA oncogenic viruses in animal model systems. The basic principles which we now apply to preparation of vaccines against lytic virus infections seem to apply as well to oncogenic viruses as tested. What we need most urgently are the proved human cancer viruses so that vaccines can be evolved for both the killed and live types.

Perkins: There is large scale production of interferon in human leucocytes using Sendai virus as an inducer.

Biggs: It would be helpful to find a naturally avirulent virus, but how would one determine that it is oncogenic?

If we find that we need a replicating virus to produce the protection associated with cell surface antigens induced by virus infection - how do we isolate these antigens? There may be, as already mentioned by Hilleman, great difficulties in their purification.

Hilleman: In response to Dr. Biggs' question, one has to find an animal model in which the animal is as sensitive to induction of cancer by the virulent virus as is man. There are situations in which such a parallel has been shown between two animal species. One might also be able to use indirect laboratory test methods to prove safety of live vaccines such as cell transformation in cell culture.

Pereira: As regards the advantages and disadvantages of the use of subunit vaccines: We shall list some of them:

1. Elimination of surplus materials from vaccines is an advantage. This applies to both nucleic acids and proteins. In the case of adenovirus, which is potentially oncogenic, the mere inactivation of viral infectivity is not sufficient *per se* to eliminate the ability of this virus to transform cells, this has been shown in a number of cases. Elimination from this vaccine of both superfluous proteins and nucleic acids is of great advantage.

2. The use of subunit vaccines permits the administration of increased doses. With crude vaccines one cannot go beyond levels, because the vaccine then begins to be toxic. In addition, the use of several highly purified antigens may allow us to produce multivalent vaccines to an extent that is not possible with crude preparations.

3. The use of purified vaccines is of advantage in enabling their standardization to be carried out by both chemical and biological methods. One can measure protein content in the purified subunit

virus and thus it would be easy to standardize the vaccine by chemical methods. Even when the vaccine is not a subunit vaccine, one is in a position to use chemical standardization, e.g., in influenza vaccines by electrophoretic methods.

4. The use of highly purified subunit vaccines solves the question of substrate where the virus is propagated. I would personally prefer to receive a crystalline virus protein vaccine produced in HeLa cells than any of a lot of crude vaccines produced in different "safe" cells.

Brunell: Ideally, one would like to have a vaccine that produces durable immunity. Could one expect to produce durable immunity with a nonreplicating vaccine as has been done with live vaccines? Could one expect to stimulate cellular immunity as well as humoral immunity with purified subunit vaccines? Are both types of immunity necessary for resistance against viral infections?

Pereira: When we compare purified vs. crude vaccine, we speak of course of killed virus vaccines. No comparison is made between live virus vaccines and subunit vaccines.

As to which cells are involved and what is the importance of humoral or cellular immunity, as a whole the question is important, but, except in a few systems, has yet to be studied.

Sela: Within the context of present-day knowledge and present-day fashions in immunology, live, attenuated virus vaccines do better than killed vaccines, chemical subunits or synthetic vaccines. If we compare, however, the killed virus vaccines with purified subunit vaccines or with the completely synthetic approaches to vaccination, there is hope that these latter may become a reality in the not too distant future. We shall have many problems pertinent to the relative importance for immunization of B and T cells, of humoral and cellular response. It will become a bioengineering problem: we can select conditions to obtain the desirable reactions, be it by aggregation or by choosing the right carrier.

Speaking about B and T cells, even their very definition is not clear. It depends on whether one uses the terminology of the sixties or of the seventies. Originally, these terms were derived from studies on chickens. T was the thymus-derived cell, important in cellular immunity, while B were Bursa-derived cells connected with humoral immunity. Nobody has yet found the precise equivalent of Bursa in man. Later, the T and B cells became known as thymus-derived cells and bone marrow-derived cells. A theory was proposed indicating that both elements are required for humoral immunity, but although we have good evidence that fits this concept of B and T cell cooperation in immune response, let us not forget that only when facts disprove a theory, the theory is disproved, but when facts agree with theory, the theory is not proved yet.

Hilleman: The relationship between antibody response to vaccination and protective immunity in influenza has thus far been shown only for whole virus vaccine. Such a relationship has not been demonstrated to date for subunit vaccines and until it is done, one cannot be assured of protective effectiveness. Dr. Norrby, I believe, showed that subunit measles vaccine was not protective, in spite of inducing antibody, while killed whole virus vaccine was effective in preventing the disease.

Pereira: We are planning to do experiments in humans with subunit vaccines and hopefully, this will give us an answer about their efficacy. Preliminary tests with ferrets, which are very difficult to protect with whole virus vaccines against influenza, are very encouraging. The subunit vaccines protect them against challenge.

Laver: One should be careful when using the term "subunit vaccines": sometimes the term is used for vaccines that are just made of components of disrupted virus and contain all sorts of elements.

Question: How does one persuade manufacturers to produce vaccines containing pure virus subunits?

Pereira: One might convince manufacturers by showing that: (a) one can increase the vaccine dose without toxic effect; (b) the subunit vaccine is much more efficient, and (c) that smaller doses may be effective.

Hilleman: The matter of persuading manufacturers is not the issue. The manufacturers will pursue what is best. One real issue is the matter of whether subunit vaccines will actually protect -- and this remains to be determined. The other real issue is cost, since people need to be able to afford what is offered them. Given two vaccines of equal efficacy and no significant adverse effects, the cheaper will be the one which is used. These practical decisions are made in the market place and quite outside the area of academic prejudices.

Sela: Before we get immunogenicity improved, let us define it. It is the capacity for triggering an immune response, be it humoral or cellular, and it is different from antigenicity which involves (a) either triggering an immune response, or (b) reacting immunospecifically with an antibody*. Thus, for example, pneumococcal polysaccharide or *B. anthrax* polyglutamic acid are not immunogenic *per se*, but react very well with antibody prepared by the complete

* Sela, Science 166:1365, 1969.

bacterium.

If the notion "immunogenicity" does not entail the notion of specificity, then while discussing immunogenicity one should discuss all the possible specificities. One should not talk about one region in the antigenic molecule as being more immunogenic than other regions; we should speak about some regions being more immunopotent than others. It seems to me that when virologists talk about immunogenicity, they mean something otherwise: when they say that this vaccine is more immunogenic they mean that it gives better protection. They would not call a cancer vaccine producing enhancing antibodies that speed up the development of a tumor an immunogenic one.

To me, the definition of immunogenicity entails the eliciting of any kind of immune response by a particular molecule. When the viral immunologists speak of immunogenicity, they mean enhancing the production of those antibodies that fight the infection. Now, one should remember that the definition of immunogenicity is operational, depending on the genetic makeup and the previous immunologic history (tolerance, paralysis). A point which has been eluded is the area of antigenic competition. It may be competition among various antigenic determinants on the same molecule or among different molecules or between two large entities. Practically, it means how many vaccines one can give at the same time and produce successful immunity. We know that when we inject serum containing some 100 different proteins, we get at best significant titers of antibodies against 30 different protein components. Is it then better to have more different determinants on the same molecule or to have a mixture of different molecules? I do not know the answer, but the question should be raised.

Adjuvanticity

Let us discuss adjuvants, such as endotoxins, pertussis or complete Freund's adjuvant. Here, as molecular immunologists, we are guilty of a grave sin: we take macromolecules known in the greatest detail, describe them atom by atom, and then we mention, paranthetically, that we study them immunologically while they are plunged in a mayonnaise containing mycobacteria. The great miracle is that the denaturation that must occur in such adjuvant mixtures, because of the lipid - water interfaces and surface inactivation, does not affect the production of good antibodies against the native protein. This is a mystery which has not yet been investigated. It is against the basic notions of a protein chemist, but it works.

As we have heard, there is still a problem with finding the right adjuvants for use in humans: when one uses incomplete Freund's adjuvant, the question remains as to the use of mineral or vegetable oil. Perhaps a non-metabolizable lecithin analogue* tied chemically to antigens would be the solution.

Synthetic Approach

My contact with immunology started with the attempt to distinguish between antigenicity and immunogenicity. We showed that we could increase the immunogenicity of gelatin, but not its specificity, by attaching to it some molecules of tyrosine**. This has been widely employed in a number of systems. For example, dextran, which is immunogenic in mice and man, is not immunogenic in rabbits. When, however, one attaches chemically a few tyrosine molecules to it, one gets excellent antibodies***. One can also introduce to non-immunogenic molecules some fatty acid chains (lauryl chains) and make non-antigenic molecules immunogenic****. Another example: when one takes a non-antigenic polymer and attaches to it sugar, it is still non-immunogenic, but when tyrosine is added, the molecule becomes immunogenic and the resulting antibodies are produced against sugar*****. The use of lauryl chains in such systems is an example of a built-in adjuvant. Still another example from Westphal's laboratory: in a *Salmonella typhi* strain there is an immunodominant character in O-acetylabequose. When one attaches this O-acetylabequose to a synthetic antigen and immunizes with it, one produces antibodies that agglutinate the whole bacterium. We do not know yet, however, what happens with the infectivity of the bacterium.

To sum up the synthetic approach: we need to attach the right antigenic specificity determinant to the genetically and immunogenetically right carrier, add the right adjuvant, and have the right metabolism to obtain optimal immune response.

Question:

Dr. Gresser, is interferon a non-specific stimulator of antibody response: Is it involved in any intermediate stage of immune response?

---

* Eibl and Westphal, Ann. 738:161, 1967.

** Arnon and Sela, Biochem. J. 75:103, 1960.

*** Sorg *et al*, Eur. J. Biochem. 17:85,1970.

**** Rüde *et al*, Eur. J. Imm. 1:113, 1971.

***** Rüde *et al*, Immunochemistry 3:137, 1966.

Gresser: As to the interaction of interferon with immune response, when one incubates sensitized lymphocytes with interferon, one enhances cell toxicity of these lymphocytes for target tumor cells. Thus in one system interferon enhances a specific activity of lymphocytes. We are currently investigating other interactions between interferon and lymphocytes.

Kohn: Referring to tyrosination techniques: Together with Fuchs we tried to attach tyrosine to killed NDV and immunize with it chickens possessing maternal antibodies. We found that the immunity achieved was not different from that obtained with a non-modified virus. I would, therefore, think that the virus *per se* is too large a complex for tyrosination and it was perhaps exaggerated to expect that it would change its immunogenicity.

Hilleman: May I comment of the practical aspects of adjuvants. There are many different kinds, of which the most effective and active are the emulsified oil adjuvants. Freund's mineral oil adjuvant has given problems in causing local reactions, probably due to the very slow metabolic removal, if any, of the mineral oil. We developed an emulsified oil adjuvant in our laboratories called adjuvant-65 which consists of components, all of which are readily metabolizable: peanut oil, Arlacel A emulsifier, and aluminum monostearate stabilizer. Such adjuvant, used with aqueous influenza vaccine, caused very good enhancement of antibody response (4 - 16-fold) as compared with the aqueous vaccine and such elevated antibody titer persists for at least six years. The dose of viral antigen may be drastically reduced - only a single dose is needed - and the antibody response is so broadened that the minor antigenic variations in influenza A which occur in the interpandemic periods are of no practical importance. The broadening of antigenic responses may, in fact, be so great as to cross pandemic virus eras. The 1957 formula vaccine in adjuvant 65, for example, gave antibody responses in 50 percent of persons to the new Hong Kong variant of 1958 whereas the aqueous vaccine gave none.

Adjuvant-65 does not cause local or systemic reactions in man. We can now, however, make chemically pure synthetic isomannide monooleate and aluminum monostearate and these are being substituted in what we call adjuvant 65-4 for the corresponding older components.

The one deterrent, to date, to licensure of adjuvant 65 in the U.S.A. has been the appearance of sarcomatous tumors in a particular breed of mice of a particular sex given the material subcutaneously. Such a phenomenon is common to rodent species following injection of a variety of irritants. The components of adjuvant 65 are not carcinogenic substances and the tumors which appear are the likely result of physico-chemical changes which, to date, have not been found to have relevance to higher species such as monkeys and man.

In reply to the question on alginates, these are not good adjuvants and introduced the problems of accumulation and sensitization.

Cabasso: In our approach to oily adjuvants, we tried to work on the principle that the less components they contained the fewer problems they presented. We, therefore, omitted emulsifiers, and used only peanut oil and aluminum monostearate.

Hilleman: It is true that one can make emulsions of aqueous vaccine with peanut oil and aluminum monostearate, but the problem is one of stability. Such vaccines must have a shelf life of at least 18 months to be practical and Arlacel A (isomannide monooleate) provides such stability.

LIST OF PARTICIPANTS

ADLER, ALISA
Hadassah Hospital, Tel-Aviv, Israel
AKOV, YAIR
Israel Institute for Biological Research, Ness-Ziona, Israel
ARNON, RUTH
Weizmann Institute of Science, Rehovot, Israel
AVTALION, RAMY
Bar-Ilan University, Ramat Gan, Israel
BARZILAI, ERGA
Kimron Veterinary Institute, Beit-Dagan, Israel
BARZILAI, ROY
Hebrew University-Hadassah Medical School, Jerusalem, Israel
BATEMAN, JOHN B.
European Research Office, London, England
BEALE, JOHN A.
The Wellcome Research Laboratories, Beckenham, Kent, England
BECKER, YECHIEL
Hebrew University-Hadassah Medical School, Jerusalem, Israel
BEEMER, ABRAHAM M.
Israel Institute for Biological Research, Ness-Ziona, Israel
BEN-DAVID, AMNON
Medical Corps, Israel Defence Forces
BEN-EFRAIM SHLOMO
Tel-Aviv University, Ramat-Aviv, Israel
BEN-PORATH, EDNA
Aba Khushy School of Medicine, Haifa, Israel
BERDICEVSKY, ISRAELA
Aba Khushy School of Medicine, Haifa, Israel
BIGGS, PETER
Houghton Poultry Research Station, Houghton, Huntingdon, England
BIRNBAUM, SHMUEL
Israel Institute for Biological Research, Ness-Ziona, Israel
BLUMENKRANTZ, RAYA
Kimron Veterinary Institute, Beit-Dagan, Israel
BORS, NETTY
Technion, Israel Institute of Technology, Haifa, Israel

BRAND, GABRIELA
Israel Institute for Biological Research, Ness-Ziona, Israel
BROTMAN, ERWIN H.
Mall Medical Group, Winnipeg, Canada
BROWN, FRED
Research Institute, Animal Virus Diseases, Pirbright, Surrey, England
BRUNELL, PHILIP
Clinical Research Centre, Harrow, Middlesex, England
CABASSO, VICTOR
Cutter Laboratories, Berkeley, California, U.S.A.
CITRI, NATHAN
Hebrew University-Hadassah Medical School, Jerusalem, Israel
COCKBURN, CHARLES W.
World Health Organization, Geneva, Switzerland
COHEN, IRUN R.
Weizmann Institute of Science, Rehovot, Israel
COHEN, NAPHTALI
District Health Office, Ministry of Health, Tel-Aviv, Israel
CYMBALISTA, SAMUEL
Microbiological Associates of Israel, Ltd., Jerusalem, Israel
DISKIN, BLUMA
Israel Institute for Biological Research, Ness-Ziona, Israel
EGOZ, NACHUM
Medical Corps, Israel Defence Forces
EVENCHIK, ZIGMUND
Israel Institute for Biological Research, Ness-Ziona, Israel
EYLAN, EMANUEL
Tel-Aviv University, Ramat-Aviv, Israel
FAINARU, MENAHEM
Weizmann Institute of Science, Rehovot, Israel
FENNER, FRANK
John Curtin School of Medical Research, Canberra, Australia
FOGEL, ALISA
Virus Laboratory, Ministry of Health, Jaffa, Israel
FUCHS, PINHAS
Israel Institute for Biological Research, Ness-Ziona, Israel
GERICHTER, CHAIM
Government Central Laboratories, Ministry of Health, Jerusalem, Israel
GINSBURG, HAIM
Weizmann Institute of Science, Rehovot, Israel
GITELMAN, JANINA
Israel Institute for Biological Research, Ness-Ziona, Israel
GOLDBLUM, NATAN
Hebrew University-Hadassah Medical School, Jerusalem, Israel
GOLDSCHMIDT, EMANUELA
Aba Khoushy School of Medicine, Haifa, Israel

GOLDSMIT, LEA
Kimron Veterinary Institute, Beit-Dagan, Israel
GOLDWASSER, ROBERT A.
Israel Institute for Biological Research, Ness-Ziona, Israel
GORDIN, MENACHEM
Hebrew University-Hadassah Medical School, Jerusalem, Israel
GORDON, ZAHAVA
Sick Fund Central Laboratory, Haifa, Israel
GOTLIEB-STEIMATZKY, TAMAR
Virus Laboratory, Ministry of Health, Jaffa, Israel
GREENBLATT, CHARLES
Hebrew University-Hadassah Medical School, Jerusalem, Israel
GRESSER, ION
Institut de Recherches sur le Cancer, Villejuif, France
GROSSMAN, ZAHAVA
Israel Institute for Biological Research, Ness-Ziona, Israel
GULIANKA, MARIANA
Kimron Veterinary Institute, Beit-Dagan, Israel
GUTTER, BEZALEL
Hebrew University-Hadassah Medical School, Jerusalem, Israel
HALEVY, MENACHEM
Israel Institute for Biological Research, Ness-Ziona, Israel
HAREL, SARA
Aba Khoushy School of Medicine, Haifa, Israel
HAY, JACOB
Israel Institute for Biological Research, Ness-Ziona, Israel
HENIG, ELIEZER
Beilinson Hospital, Petah Tikva, Israel
HERTMAN, ISRAEL
Israel Institute for Biological Research, Ness-Ziona, Israel
HERZBERG, HANNA
Israel Institute for Biological Research, Ness-Ziona, Israel
HILLEMAN, MAURICE R.
Merck, Sharp & Dohme Research Laboratories, West Point, Pa., U.S.A.
HORNSTEIN, LEA
Sick Fund Central Laboratory, Haifa, Israel
IANCONESCU, MARIUS
Kimron Veterinary Institute, Beit-Dagan, Israel
ISRAELI, EYTAN
Israel Institute for Biological Research, Ness-Ziona, Israel
KALMAR, ELIZABETH
Kimron Veterinary Institute, Beit-Dagan, Israel
KATZ, DAVID
Israel Institute for Biological Research, Ness-Ziona, Israel
KATZ, EHUD
Hebrew University-Hadassah Medical School, Jerusalem, Israel
KAYE, MYRA
Israel Institute for Biological Research, Ness-Ziona, Israel

KEYSARY, AVI
Israel Institute for Biological Research, Ness-Ziona, Israel
KINAMON, SIMHA
Ministry of Defence, Israel
KIRCHSTEIN, RUTH
National Institutes of Health, Bethesda, Maryland, U.S.A.
KLINGBERG, MARCUS A.
Israel Institute for Biological Research, Ness-Ziona, Israel
KLINGBERG, WANDA
Israel Institute for Biological Research, Ness-Ziona, Israel
KLEINBERG, DANIELA
Israel Institute for Biological Research, Ness-Ziona, Israel
KOHN, ALEXANDER
Israel Institute for Biological Research, Ness-Ziona, Israel
KOHN, CHANA
Sick Fund Central Laboratory, Rehovot, Israel
KOT, YEHUDA
Technion, Israel Institute of Technology, Haifa, Israel
KUTTIN, ELIEZER S.
Israel Institute for Biological Research, Ness-Ziona, Israel
LACHMI, BATEL
Hebrew University-Hadassah Medical School, Jerusalem
LAHAV, MIRA
Sick Fund Central Laboratory, Tel-Aviv, Israel
LARON, DORA
Virus Laboratory, Ministry of Health, Jaffa, Israel
LAVER, W.G.
John Curtin School of Medical Research, Canberra, Australia
LERCHE, CHRISTIAN
National Institute of Public Health, Oslo, Norway
LEV,RAN
Israel Defence Forces
LEVANON, AVIGDOR
Israel Institute for Biological Research, Ness-Ziona, Israel
LEVENTON-KRISS, SOPHIE
Virus Laboratory, Ministry of Health, Jaffa, Israel
LEVI, MAURICE
Haifa, Israel
LEVINE, PINCUS P.
New York State Veterinary College, Ithaca, New York, U.S.A.
LEVISOHN, SHARON
Kimron Veterinary Institute, Beit-Dagan, Israel
LEVY, EMMANUEL
Central Emek Hospital, Afula, Israel
LEVY, REUVEN
Hebrew University-Hadassah Medical School, Jerusalem, Israel
MALKINSON, MERTYN
Kimron Veterinary Institute, Beit-Dagan, Israel

MANOR, DAPHNA
Hebrew University-Hadassah Medical School, Jerusalem, Israel
MANSON, LIONEL A.
The Wistar Institute, Philadelphia, Pa., U.S.A.
MARINOV, URI
National Council for Research and Development, Jerusalem, Israel
MARKENSON, JACOB
Israel Institute for Biological Research, Ness-Ziona, Israel
MARZOUK, JOSEPH
Virus Laboratory, Ministry of Health, Jaffa, Israel
MATES, ABRAHAM
Bar-Ilan University, Ramat-Gan, Israel
MERDINGER, MOSHE
Kimron Veterinary Institute, Beit-Dagan, Israel
MERZBACH, DAVID
Aba Khoushy School of Medicine, Haifa, Israel
MICHAEL, AMNON
Vineland Laboratories Ltd., Kfar Vitkin, Israel
MICHAELI, DAN
Medical Corps, Israel Defence Forces
MILLER, GEORGE
Israel Institute for Biological Research, Ness-Ziona, Israel
MISKIN, ABRAHAM
Kaplan Hospital, Rehovot, Israel
MIZRAHI, AVSHALOM
Israel Institute for Biological Research, Ness-Ziona, Israel
MOZES, EDNA
Weizmann Institute of Science, Rehovot, Israel
MUHSAM, BRURIA
Hebrew University-Hadassah Medical School, Jerusalem, Israel
NAGAN, LEHAIM
Medical Corps, Israel Defence Forces
NIR, YEHUDA
Israel Institute for Biological Research, Ness-Ziona, Israel
NISHMI, MOSHE
Hebrew University-Hadassah Medical School, Jerusalem, Israel
NORRBY, ERLING
Karolinska Institute, Stockholm, Sweden
OFEK, ITZHAK
Government Central Laboratories, Jerusalem, Israel
OLSHEWSKY, UDI
Hebrew University-Hadassah Medical School, Jerusalem, Israel
OMLAND, TOV
National Institute of Public Health, Oslo, Norway
OREN, RACHEL
Israel Institute for Biological Research, Ness-Ziona, Israel
PAYES, BENJAMIN
Israel Institute for Biological Research, Ness-Ziona, Israel

PELEG, BEN-AMI
Kimron Veterinary Institute, Beit-Dagan, Israel
PEREIRA, HELIO G.
National Institute for Medical Research, London, England
PEREIRA, MARGARET S.
Virus Reference Laboratories, London, England
PERKINS, FRANK T.
National Institute for Medical Research, London, England
PLUZNIK, DOV
Bar-Ilan University, Ramat-Gan, Israel
PRUDOVSKY, SARA
Kimron Veterinary Institute, Beit-Dagan, Israel
RABINOWICZ, SONIA
Government Central Laboratories, Jerusalem, Israel
RAFAELI, DVORA
Aba Khoushy School of Medicine, Haifa, Israel
RANNON, LOTTE
Virus Laboratory, Ministry of Health, Jaffa, Israel
RASHI, MOSHE
Miles-Yeda Ltd., Rehovot, Israel
RAVID, ZOHAR
Hebrew University-Hadassah Medical School, Jerusalem, Israel
RAZIN, SHMUEL
Hebrew University-Hadassah Medical School, Jerusalem, Israel
ROSENKRANZ, HERBERT
Columbia University, New York, N.Y., U.S.A.
ROTEM, YAACOV
Chaim Sheba Medical Centre, Tel-Hashomer, Israel
ROTH, JESSE
Hebrew University-Hadassah Medical School, Jerusalem, Israel
ROTHFELD, MIRIAM
Sick Fund Central Laboratories, Haifa, Israel
ROZENSZAJN, ARIE
Bar-Ilan University, Ramat-Gan, Israel
SAAR, MICHAEL
Israel Institute for Biological Research, Ness-Ziona, Israel
SALOMON, FEIGA
Asaf Harofeh Government Hospital, Zrifin, Israel
SANDBERG, ORNA
Israel Institute for Biological Research, Ness-Ziona, Israel
SELA, MICHAEL
Weizmann Institute of Science, Rehovot, Israel
SHAPIRA, ADAM
Israel Institute for Biological Research, Ness-Ziona, Israel
SHAPIRA-HIRSCH, RAYA
Sick Fund Central Laboratory, Haifa, Israel
SHENBERG, ESTHER
Israel Institute for Biological Research, Ness-Ziona, Israel

SINAI, JUDITH
Israel Institute for Biological Research, Ness-Ziona, Israel
SKALSKY, PAULINA
Virus Laboratory, Ministry of Health, Jaffa, Israel
SOMPOLINSKY, DAVID
Bar-Ilan University, Ramat-Gan, Israel
SPIRA, DAN
Hebrew University-Hadassah Medical School, Jerusalem, Israel
SPIRA, GAD
Hebrew University-Hadassah Medical School, Jerusalem, Israel
SPIRA, NILY
Kimron Veterinary Institute, Beit-Dagan, Israel
STEIMAN, YONEL
Israel Institute for Biological Research, Ness-Ziona
STRAKS, RACHEL
Israel Institute for Biological Research, Neww-Ziona, Israel
STRAUSSMAN, YOHEVED
Israel Institute for Biological Research, Ness-Ziona, Israel
SULITZEANU, DOV
Hebrew University, Jerusalem, Israel
SZEINBERG, ARIEH
Chaim Sheba Medical Centre, Tel-Hashomer, Israel
SZEINBERG, BILHA
Chaim Sheba Medical Centre, Tel-Hashomer, Israel
SWARTZ, TIBERIO
Israel Institute for Biological Research, Ness-Ziona, Israel
TORTEN, MICHAEL
Israel Institute for Biological Research, Ness-Ziona, Israel
TRAININ, ZEEV
Kimron Veterinary Institute, Beit-Dagan, Israel
TURNER, ILANA
Israel Institute for Biological Research, Ness-Ziona, Israel
WALDMAN, ROBERT H.
University of Florida, Gainesville, Florida, U.S.A.
WHITE, MICHAEL
Vineland Laboratories Ltd., Kfar Vitkin, Israel
WINTER, SIMON
Rothschild Hospital, Haifa, Israel
WISSEMAN, CHARLES L., JR.
University of Maryland School of Medicine, Baltimore, Md., U.S.A.
YEKUTIEL, PEREZ
Tel-Aviv University Medical School, Ramat-Aviv, Israel
YOFE, JACOB
Jerusalem, Israel
YORAV, HANOCH
Israel Institute for Biological Research, Ness-Ziona, Israel

ZAKAY-RONES, ZICHRIA
Hebrew University-Hadassah Medical School, Jerusalem, Israel
ZUCKERMAN, AVIVAH
Hebrew University, Jerusalem, Israel
ZYDON, YAACOV
Israel Institute for Biological Research, Ness-Ziona, Israel
ZYLBER, ESTHER
Hebrew University-Hadassah Medical School, Jerusalem, Israel

SUBJECT INDEX

GPSR Compliance
The European Union's (EU) General Product Safety Regulation (GPSR) is a set of rules that requires consumer products to be safe and our obligations to ensure this.

If you have any concerns about our products, you can contact us on

ProductSafety@springernature.com

In case Publisher is established outside the EU, the EU authorized representative is:

Springer Nature Customer Service Center GmbH
Europaplatz 3
69115 Heidelberg, Germany

www.ingramcontent.com/pod-product-compliance
Ingram Content Group UK Ltd.
Pitfield, Milton Keynes, MK11 3LW, UK
UKHW051130260726
13967UKWH00010B/2966